Embracing
LIFE
Great Comebacks
from Ostomy Surgery

Embracing
LIFE

Great Comebacks
from Ostomy Surgery

The inspirational stories
of twelve people who have
survived and thrived
following ostomy surgery.

by
ROLF BENIRSCHKE
with Elaine Minamide

Rolf Benirschke Enterprises
San Diego, California

Embracing Life: Great Comebacks from Ostomy Surgery
by Rolf Benirschke with Elaine Minamide
© 2009 Rolf Benirschke Enterprises, Inc.
All rights reserved.

FIRST EDITION

ISBN 978-0-9720065-1-4

Cover and back photos: Greg Schneider

Cover and interior design: Michael Loftus · Loftus Design Associates

Printed in the United States of America

Table of Contents

Acknowledgments

Foreword
by Victor Fazio, M.D.,
Chairman of the Department of Colon-Rectal Surgery
at the Cleveland Clinic

Dedication

To everyone facing ostomy surgery . . .
and to their family, friends, surgeons,
and wound and ostomy nurses
who will help them get through
this life-saving procedure.

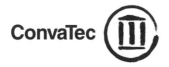

ConvaTec

David I. Johnson
CEO
200 Headquarters Park Drive
Skillman, New Jersey, 08558
Phone: 908.904.2500

On behalf of ConvaTec, a leading developer and marketer of innovative medical technologies that have helped improve the lives of millions of people worldwide, it is my pleasure to present you with this copy of *Embracing LIFE*, by Rolf Benirschke, an NFL legend, a colitis patient and a person who has lived with an ostomy.

This book was inspired by Rolf's own true life story and his painful battle with ulcerative colitis. Following his ostomy surgery, as he fought to return to the game he loved he became acutely aware that there were thousands of others engaged in the same battle and, in the process, he discovered his life mission.

In 1984, Rolf founded the Great Comebacks® Program, a patient support network that provides guidance and inspiration for people facing the physical and emotional challenges of Crohn's disease, ulcerative colitis, colorectal cancer and ostomy surgery. It was his belief that, by uncovering and sharing stories from other patients who had successfully overcome ostomy surgery and returned to a normal and fulfilling life, he could encourage and inspire others to keep fighting.

As a co-sponsor of the Great Comebacks Program, we at ConvaTec draw inspiration from Rolf and the remarkable individuals profiled in *Embracing LIFE* who light the way for thousands of other people with intestinal diseases and their families by showing that the world – far from being an isolated, lonely place – is brimming with possibilities. They teach us so much about personal courage and perseverance, and inspire all of us at ConvaTec every day to develop new technologies and provide support for people having ostomy surgery.

I hope you enjoy *Embracing LIFE*, and trust you will find it as inspirational and encouraging as I did. If you would like to learn more about Rolf's story, I also encourage you to pick up a copy of his autobiography, *Alive & Kicking*.

All of us at ConvaTec want to wish you all the best.

Sincerely,

David I. Johnson
CEO

Acknowledgements

Writing books like *Alive & Kicking*, *Great Comebacks from Ostomy Surgery*, and *Embracing Life* as well as speaking around the country to doctors, nurses, and patients about what it takes to come back from ostomy surgery has been a passion of mine ever since I was forced to recover from my own ostomy surgery back in 1979.

That was a difficult time for me because I was young and just beginning my career as a professional athlete. I had always been healthy, perhaps taking my health for granted, and things like that just weren't supposed to happen . . . at least that was my thinking at the time.

But ostomy surgeries *do* happen, and each year there are approximately 130,000 such surgeries performed in the United States alone . . . and many to young people. From my own experiences, I know that each operation is life-changing for the patient and his or her family. Each one of us goes through the same feelings of anger, self-doubt, frustration, and fear about the future.

I was privileged to be the placekicker for the San Diego Chargers when I went through my illness, living in a city where our professional football team was adored by the community. As a member of that team, I received hundreds of letters from fans and know that I was prayed for and encouraged in every way a fan could possibly support a player. I recognize that not everyone is so fortunate, and that most people are forced to go through their trials alone or with little encouragement from those around them.

Embracing Life is written with the idea that if a new patient could read about how other individuals—young and old, male and female, athletic and not—describe what it was like to go through their ostomy surgeries, then we would have a book that would be an encouragement for others. With that goal in mind, and with the help of wound, ostomy and continence nurses, colon and rectal surgeons, and patients I have met over the years, I have assembled a special collection of stories that should be a valuable resource for any new patients facing ostomy surgery.

The completion of *Embracing Life* would not be possible without the support and encouragement from the volunteers at the Crohn's & Colitis Foundation of America, the United Ostomy Associations of America, and the people I have the good fortune of working with at ConvaTec.

Since the company was founded in 1978, ConvaTec's commitment to its patients has been unwavering and has propelled it to become the world leader in the manufacture and distribution of wound and ostomy supplies. I consider it a privilege to work alongside ConvaTec and their dedicated employees to help raise the awareness of ostomy surgery and to educate and encourage doctors, nurses, and patients around the world.

Although I'm convinced this book will inspire anyone who reads it, I'm reminded that the decision to get "better" and not stay "bitter" is still up to each one of us . . . and it *is* a decision. When I was playing in the NFL, we had top-notch coaches preparing us each week. When Game Day rolled around, however, and the players stepped on to the field of play, the outcome was up to us. Winning or losing was determined by how well we performed individually and as a team, and how well we executed the game plan we had been taught.

And so it is with ostomy surgery. After reading this book, I hope you'll come away with the understanding that while your circumstances may seem brutally unfair at times, that's life. What becomes most important is how you confront your situation. In

Embracing Life, you will hear from remarkable people who have gone through horrific medical experiences, but who have each made the decision not to let their circumstances control their outcomes or keep them from doing the things they were most passionate about.

When you make a similar decision, you have the opportunity to discover the amazing indomitable human spirit that God has gifted each one of us with. You will learn that you have a greater ability to cope, possess more courage and perseverance than you ever imagined, and have a chance to use very difficult circumstances to completely transform your life and turn what seems like a bleak medical situation into an amazing blessing . . . but it is up to you.

I hope you enjoy *Embracing Life* as much as I did compiling this book. May you find great inspiration from these special individuals who "got real" to show others the way and to provide hope that things really can work out . . . *if you embrace life.*

Rolf Benirschke

Foreword

by Victor Fazio, M.D.

*Chairman of the Department of Colon-Rectal Surgery
at the Cleveland Clinic*

Several years ago, Rolf Benirschke asked me to write the Foreword for *Great Comebacks from Ostomy Surgery*, and I readily agreed. What a great resource for ostomy patients! I must have handed out hundreds of copies, and I know that the special collection of compelling stories from actual patients helped lift the spirits of my patients and gave them the encouragement and inspiration they needed in their fight to get their lives back.

Now, Rolf has come out with *Embracing Life: Great Comebacks from Ostomy Surgery*, another book of remarkable stories. The folks you are about to meet come from all walks of life, but they have one thing in common: an unyielding desire to not only survive ostomy surgery but to get back and return to doing what they are passionate about.

Perhaps you're holding this book because you're dealing with a severe case of Crohn's disease or ulcerative colitis, or perhaps you just went through cancer surgery. You're unsure about the future, fearful of the unknown. You've heard your doctor mention the possibility of ostomy surgery, but you don't know if you can handle that. But you're sick and tired of the interminable diarrhea, the horrible abdominal cramps, and the uncontrollable need to go at the most inopportune moments.

Perhaps the thought of wearing an appliance to collect your waste sounds like a fate worse than death. I wouldn't blame you if you felt that like. I've met thousands of patients just like you. You've withstood years of physical discomfort and pain, and you've done everything possible to avoid surgery. But now you're at the end of the line, and you understand that ostomy surgery may now be your last option.

It makes me sad to think of what people like you have gone through. Not just you but your parents, your children, and your friends. I'm sad because I know it doesn't have to be that way . . . and shouldn't be that way. You see, I have performed more than 5,000 ostomy surgeries since 1973, and the almost universal reaction I receive soon after the operation is, "Doctor, if I had only known I was going to feel this good, I never would have waited so long."

Now instead of having to convince patients on my own, I can just hand them a copy of *Embracing Life: Great Comebacks from Ostomy Surgery*. It's great to have a resource that can help patients get the answers and be inspired at the same time . . . by people who've been there.

Victor W. Fazio, M.D., is chairman of the Department of Colorectal Surgery and vice-chairman of the Division of Surgery at The Cleveland Clinic in Cleveland, Ohio. He has held both positions for twenty-five years. Board-certified in colon and rectal surgery, Dr. Fazio's clinical interests are Crohn's disease and ulcerative colitis, colorectal cancer, and pelvic floor reservoir procedures for ulcerative colitis and familial polyposis.

Dr. Fazio was awarded the Premier Physician Award from the Crohn's & Colitis Foundation in 1992. Under his co-direction, treatment for digestive diseases at The Cleveland Clinic is ranked second in the country in U.S. News & World Report's annual survey of top hospitals. In 2000, he was the first recipient of The Cleveland Clinic Master Clinician Award.

A frequent lecturer at national and international medical meetings, Dr. Fazio has authored more than 500 scientific papers on surgical treatment for colorectal cancers, as well as ostomy management. He has also written seven books on what he has learned in the surgical bay over the years.

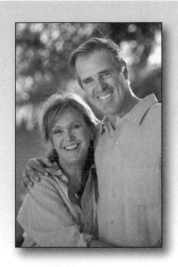

Rolf Benirschke

AGE: 53

HOMETOWN: San Diego, California

MEDICAL SITUATION:
In his second season as the placekicker for the San Diego Chargers, Rolf became sick with inflammatory bowel disease and would need life-saving ostomy surgery at the age of twenty-four—but what about his NFL career?

"**R**olf, we need to know more. I'm scheduling you for a colonoscopy tomorrow. A visual exam should help us make the diagnosis more conclusive," announced my physician.

The idea that my doctor would insert a long metal instrument up my rectum and into my colon to see whether there was inflammation or ulcerations on the colon's lining sounded painful and perhaps the most humiliating medical test a human being could be asked to endure.

How had it all come to this? I was twenty-four years old, and before the diarrhea and abdominal spasms started, I had been in great health. I had to be, after all, I was a professional athlete—the placekicker for the San Diego Chargers. I was in my second season with the team and was earning a reputation as one of the league's most accurate young kickers. For several weeks, however, I had struggled with severe abdominal cramps, bloody diarrhea, and a persistent fever. My doctor initially prescribed prednisone (a powerful anti-inflammatory corticosteroid drug) and Azulfidine (an anti-bacterial drug), but my condition failed to improve. Suspecting that I might have Crohn's disease, he decided that I needed a colonoscopy to find out for sure.

The day of the procedure was a memorable one. After checking in with the nurse, I was handed a hospital gown, told to change, and then directed to lie face down on the examining table. If you have ever worn one of those gowns, then you know how hard it is to preserve any sense of modesty. I felt as though my backside was open for the whole world to see.

"So, this is what a professional football player looks like," the nurse joked, trying to be clever as she readied me for the procedure. I was in no mood for humor, however, and gritted my teeth until I was given the mild anesthetic. Although I couldn't feel much, I had a vague sensation that I was being "plumbed" by an invasive device traveling up way too far. Let's just say the scoping procedure will never be on my "Top Ten" list of fun things to do.

Despite the "view" and biopsy, my physicians were still unable to confirm a diagnosis other than to say that I had inflammatory bowel disease (IBD). They were fairly confident that I had Crohn's disease but could not rule out ulcerative colitis. I would later learn that almost one-and-a-half million people in the United States suffer from IBD and that approximately 15 percent of those cases can't be conclusively diagnosed either. (I would live under the impression that I had Crohn's disease for four years before finding out that it was actually ulcerative colitis that I had been suffering from all along.)

Despite the best efforts of my doctors, my health continued to deteriorate. Although I was able to keep playing during the 1978 NFL football season, I was steadily losing weight and strength. By midseason, I was no longer strong enough to kick off effectively, although I continued to kick field goals and extra points. Things got worse during the last month of the season.

Eating caused terrible pain and horrible cramping each time my severely inflamed gut received food, so I basically stopped eating. I needed nutrition to perform on the football field, however, so my doctors decided that I should be fed intravenously. In this way, my body would receive enough calories while my bowels would receive a rest.

I settled into the following routine: kick during Sunday's game, check into the hospital Sunday night, and have a central total parental nutritional (TPN) line inserted into my jugular vein in my neck, from which I would receive "liquid food" all week. On Saturday, I would be released from the hospital to join the team's road trip or spend the night locally at the Charger's team hotel prior to Sunday's home game. Following the final whistle, I would once again check myself into the hospital and get hooked back up to the TPN line. The only physical exercise I was allowed during the week were the "laps" I could make around the hospital halls.

Looking back on all this, I realize how crazy this schedule sounds. But remember, in my mind and to others around me, I had a bad "stomach ache" and a touch of diarrhea. Pro football players learn to play with pain; after all, this was the NFL, where my teammates were separating shoulders, tearing up knees, and sustaining all kinds of other "real" injuries, yet they continued to play on Game Day.

But there was another motivation to endure the weeklong IV feedings and hospital stays. I was scared . . . frightened to death. I was scared that the awful pain would never go away. That I would spend the rest of my life needing to know where every bathroom was and that I would never be healthy again. My life was flashing before me, and I didn't like what I was seeing.

I was also scared that I might lose my job. I loved being an NFL kicker. I loved the competition and the fact that people were counting on me. I loved that my kicks often had a big impact on the outcome of a game. Playing in the NFL was exciting, and I didn't want to give it up or let some rotten disease take that experience away from me. You see, in professional football there is room for only one kicker on a team. You were either playing every Sunday, or you were bounced out of the league. I knew that if I were forced to take some time off, I would be replaced and probably lose my job. Those thoughts petrified me, so I endured. I kept my thoughts and fears to myself and carried on . . . trying desperately to make it to the end of the season.

The weird thing was that I continued to kick well. At one point, I hit sixteen consecutive field goals, and under our new coach Don Coryell and quarterback Dan Fouts, the team was really coming together. We wouldn't make it to the playoffs that year, but we did make life miserable for a bunch of other teams trying to get there.

Somehow I made it through the 1978 season without missing a game. While things were looking up for the Chargers, my future was increasingly uncertain.

One Sick Puppy

Once the season was over, I knew I had to find a way to try to stabilize my inflammatory bowel disease. I knew I couldn't go through another season like the one I had just endured, and I didn't want to even consider the possibility of surgery. Remember, professional football is a ruthless business where the weak and the sick are discarded. Besides, everyone felt that the Chargers would be in the playoff hunt, and I wanted to be part of the team.

Meanwhile, I was still experiencing piercing cramps, bouts of nausea, and nonstop diarrhea. I spent the entire six-month off-season reading everything I could find, learning as much as I could, and trying every treatment imaginable to get rid of the disease.

In order to keep my weight up, the team trainers and a nutritionist came up with a plan to supplement my diet with special high-caloric "milkshakes" brimming with amino acids and carbohydrates. The problem was that I had to drink *fifteen* of those vile purple-colored concoctions each day. They tasted so bad that I had to literally plug my nose in order to get them down. It was no fun, but I would do almost anything to keep kicking.

When the 1979 season opened, I had regained some of my weight and appeared to be relatively stable. At least, that is what I tried to convince myself was happening. The season started with a bang as I kicked four field goals in our opening game win over the Seattle Seahawks. We were off and running, but with each game, I realized that it was just a matter of time. Following every kick, the pain was so excruciating that I had to sit down on the bench and wait out the piercing abdominal cramps knifing through my gut.

Several weeks later, we traveled to Boston to play the New England Patriots. In pre-game warm-ups, I could barely kick a 35-yard field goal despite a stiff wind at my back. It was clear that my prolonged battle with IBD was taking its toll. How long could I hold out? How long before I would cost the team with my inability to kick a long-range field goal?

Those thoughts haunted me as I boarded the team plane following our disappointing loss to the Patriots. I was not looking forward to the long, cross-country flight home.

Not long after take-off, I began to feel feverish while intense abdominal cramps assaulted me. My world started spinning, and I must have blacked out. When I came to I was on fire—103 degrees! Despite my high temperature, my body shivered with chills. Someone alerted the team doctor, who quickly ordered my teammates to carefully lay me across three seats and wrap me in several blankets. They applied ice packs to my forehead as I shook violently with the fever that ravaged my insides.

The team doctor knew I was very sick and felt I would have to be hospitalized upon touchdown in San Diego. When we finally landed, however, I was feeling somewhat better, and I convinced my parents to take me to their house rather than to the hospital. In my mind, I still wasn't willing to give in and admit I couldn't go on any more.

Two days later, a panel of my doctors made the decision for me, however, and I was admitted to University Hospital in San Diego. My season was over just four games after it had begun, but more importantly, the inevitable had finally come to pass . . . I would need surgery. One year of debilitating diarrhea and stomach cramps had taken its toll. I was worn out. I had tried everything I knew to try, but I just couldn't fight it anymore. The disease was not in my head, as so many uninformed people had suggested, but was a real physical ailment that was not only threatening my career but also my life.

Dr. Gerald Peskin, my surgeon, explained that he would most likely perform a resection, or the removal of the diseased part of my bowel. He didn't believe I would need an ostomy, one of my deepest fears, but he had me sign consent papers nonetheless. The problem was that since I was so weak from my extended battle with the disease, he felt it would be necessary to wait two weeks while TPN feedings built up my strength.

I was feeling pretty sorry for myself as I lay in the hospital room watching my football career vanish right before my eyes. *This is not fair. This shouldn't be happening to me. Not now . . . not when the team is just getting good and my kicking career is just taking off.*

Just then one of my attending physicians came in. Dr. Cammy Mowery had impressed me with her sensitivity when we had first been introduced. Now, the pent-up fears and uncertainties came tumbling out. "Is this ever going to end?" I whined. "Am I ever going to get over this?" I was so miserable that I was sobbing.

Dr. Mowery listened quietly and seemed to understand my desperation. "You want to know the truth, Rolf? The truth is you're not the first to go through this. We have a half-dozen other people on the floor with inflammatory bowel disease right now. And across the nation, there are hundreds—make that thousands—of other people in hospitals with exactly the same thing you have. The point is your situation is not unique. I know a little bit about your background in football, and I have great confidence that you can get through this." She squeezed my hand as she comforted me.

Meanwhile, abdominal cramps continued to ravage my insides, particularly after the now-routine instances of explosive diarrhea. A blood workup revealed that I was getting toxic and indicated the presence of bacteria in my bloodstream. My doctors decided surgery could not wait, so they scheduled the operation for the following morning.

It was quite by chance, or maybe it wasn't, that Dr. Larry Saidman, the doctor who would be my anesthesiologist, stopped by that afternoon to check up on me and see whether I had any questions. When he walked into my room, he found me sprawled on the floor, passed out in the bathroom.

When I came to, sweat was beading up on my forehead and running in rivulets down the sides of my face. My hands trembled, and I had trouble focusing on his words. My body, which was experiencing severe septic shock, shook violently from the fever.

Realizing the gravity of my situation, Dr. Saidman immediately called Dr. Peskin while I was prepped before being rushed into the operating room. After some discussion, the decision was made to proceed with the resection. A twelve-inch long incision was made on my abdomen, and my ascending colon and part of my transverse colon were snipped out. The doctors then reconnected the end of my small intestine to the remaining transverse colon and stitched me back together.

I had dodged the ostomy bullet, but had no idea that my real medical problems were just beginning.

Fevers and Spikes

After any major abdominal surgery, it's critical to keep expanding the lungs to lessen the possibility of developing pneumonia. That's why I was connected to a respirator in the Intensive Care Unit, which forced me to take deep breaths.

With each heave, however, my lacerated stomach muscles screamed in pain. Shortly after arriving in the ICU, I began experiencing fever spikes. Out of nowhere, my temperature would shoot up, but my teeth would begin chattering violently while my body shook uncontrollably. It felt as though my incision was being ripped open with each shake. These episodes lasted for up to forty-five minutes, and I would lie helplessly shaking, shivering with cold on the outside, but burning up inside.

Those horrible chills and fever spikes tormented me for days. My temperature would often get up to 104 or 105 degrees—dangerously high. Only doses of morphine eased the pain; ice packs, Tylenol, and a water mattress helped control the fevers. I was a very sick young man who was fast losing hope.

The mystery behind the unexplained fevers was revealed when cultures indicated the presence of gram-negative organisms—*E. coli* bacteria in my blood. My doctors feared I had either an abscess or a leak in the suture line where the two ends of my intestine had been sewn together—a critical complication that causes people to die.

"Dr. Peskin, what's happening?" I pleaded as he stopped by on one of his twice-daily visits.

"Well, we're not exactly sure," he replied looking at my chart. "But it appears we can't wait any longer. I'm afraid that we're going to have to go back in and find out."

"You mean another surgery?" I looked at him through horrified eyes. "Are you talking about cutting me up again?"

"Rolf, there's something clearly wrong. We have no choice," Dr. Peskin answered gravely. "We have to find out what's going on and fix it."

Six days after my initial resection, Dr. Peskin and his team sliced me open once again and peered into my abdominal cavity for a second time. They quickly found the problem. A small leak at the suture line where the ileum and the colon had been reconnected had become a big gaping hole. The bacteria that normally live in my gut were now spilling into my abdomen and getting into my bloodstream, causing acute peritonitis.

"My God, look at that infection!" Dr. Peskin exclaimed to the other doctors. "I hope we caught it in time. Any longer, and the Chargers would definitely be looking for a new kicker."

The inevitable happened next—an ostomy . . . actually two ostomies. The doctors carefully snipped another inch off the end of my ileum, than began plotting where to locate the functioning ileostomy on the right side of my torso. This was where an appliance would now collect my fecal waste.

But because my surgery had been performed under emergency conditions, and because I was so sick, my doctors didn't believe I would have survived the time it would have taken to do a total colectomy, where my entire colon and rectum would have been removed.

Because of this, they were forced to create a second stoma to secure the remaining part of my colon. Rather than just leaving the rest of my large intestine to flop around inside my abdomen, they created a mucous fistula colostomy that would hold my now non-functioning colon in place. It would require a second bag to collect the epithelial cells that slough off the lining of the colon, which now served no purpose.

Normally, ostomy surgeries are well planned, and careful attention is paid to where the stomas are placed on the body. Stomas are generally located below the belt line so that the appliances are out of the way and the patient's belt does not restrict the opening.

For reasons I cannot fathom to this day, my stoma was mistakenly placed above my belt line. Perhaps the doctors weren't paying close attention because my surgery was performed under such stressful conditions, or perhaps the doctors just miscalculated. At any rate, stomas located above the belt line make for difficult lifestyle complications later.

To close me up, doctors sewed large wire sutures into the incision that started under my sternum and traveled south past my belly button to just above my pubic bone. Now that I was an ostomate, the NFL seemed like a world away.

Struggling Each Day

I was in bad shape when the nurses wheeled me back from the Recovery Room to the ICU. When I groggily came to and learned that an ostomy had been performed, I couldn't believe it. I was numb. Surely when I go back to sleep and wake up again, I'll learn that this was all just some kind of bad dream. Did they really say I had two bags?

During the few lucid moments between my drug-induced naps, I wondered whether life was actually worth fighting for. What was the point? I would never be able to kick in the NFL again. Worse, I would never again participate in the other sports and outdoor activities I loved. From where I was lying, my life was all but over. When the nurses changed my dressings for the first time and I caught a glimpse of my horribly cut-up stomach, I received visual confirmation that things were bad . . . *really* bad.

As if to make matters worse, I was seized again by shaking chills. For days the fevers raged, and my resting pulse more than doubled. I felt ice cold and begged for warm blankets. Each day was a monumental struggle. I didn't realize it at the time, but I was in a real battle for my life.

Four days after my surgery, Melba Conner, an enterostomal therapy nurse, gave me my first ileostomy lesson. Barely coherent at the time, I wasn't in the mood to deal with my ostomy. There was too much else going on to come to grips with the fact that I would now have to live with a bag.

Melba was persistent, however, and when I found out she had an ileostomy of her own, I grudgingly listened. It turned out that she had loads of experience and had actually become one of the first ET nurses in the country. She talked openly about living with an appliance, what I could expect, and how little it would change my lifestyle. Still, I was overwhelmed at everything happening to me.

"I don't know, Melba. I'm not sure I can handle all of this," I said, barely choking back tears.

"It's not a question of whether you can handle it," she stated firmly. "There is simply no option. Besides, if it weren't for the surgery, you'd be six feet under right now. Remember that always."

I stared at her. She had my attention now.

"I know this is an enormous change for anybody," she continued, "and maybe more so for someone as athletic as you. Listen, I don't follow football much, but I've never heard the nurses talk about a patient getting so much mail. You must have a lot of friends out there who really care about you, so if I were you, I'd start by being thankful for my blessings."

I nodded and continued to listen.

"Now, let's get to the basics," said Melba, as she touched my stoma with her index finger. "It's going to seem like a lot of information at first, but for now, just watch what I do."

I shook my head and closed my eyes. *If only those bags would disappear.*

"Look, Rolf," she said, as if she was reading my mind. "These appliances are not going away. You have to learn how they work. For the rest of your life, you're going to have to do this. If you learn well, they shouldn't interfere with anything you do—anything!"

Melba took my hand and had me touch my left stoma. It was shiny, a bit wet-looking, and dark pink—not unlike the lining of my mouth. The one-inch round stoma protruded from my left side about half an inch and didn't have any feeling.

Melba explained that there weren't any nerve endings in the stoma, so touching couldn't hurt. The stoma's redness meant it was well vascularized, she continued, adding that I may notice a little blood—perfectly natural and no cause for alarm—when changing the appliance.

"You're lucky to have had your surgery now and not ten years ago," she said. "Modern appliances today allow you to go four or five days before changing faceplates. They are easy on your skin, won't leak or smell, and no one has to know you are even wearing one. It wasn't so long ago that there was virtually nothing available. Patients would have to create their own appliance, using old rubber heating water bottles, cans, plastic bags, or whatever else they could come up with. They would leak and smell, and the corrosion on a person's skin was absolutely horrendous."

"Maybe I am fortunate," I said with a little optimism, and the first positive thought I'd had in a while.

"You are," she replied. "Now let's change those appliances of yours."

Melba gently removed my old appliances and cleaned around the stomas with soap and water. She was careful not to snag anything on my protruding wire sutures or touch my painful incision. Then she dried around them with a towel and used a skin prep to clean the area. Next, she cut two stoma-sized holes out of a pair of faceplate barriers that would snugly sit around the stomas to protect my skin from the burning digestive enzymes. Before she attached them, however, she spread a whitish paste around my stomas and waited several minutes for the glue to get tacky. (Paste is not necessary with nearly all of today's appliances, and changing one today takes just a moment. In fact, most faceplates now come precut or with a moldable opening that makes the entire changing process incredibly easy.)

With the gentleness of someone who had done this a thousand times before, she carefully fitted the faceplates over my stomas one at a time and pressed firmly to seal them. After adding some paper tape around the faceplate borders, she attached the new pouches and snapped them into a secure position. *Voila!* I had new appliances. The whole process took only ten minutes and seemed relatively simple.

Melba checked the clip on the bag collecting the waste. "When you're up and around, you're going to need to empty your pouch six or seven times a day, depending on how much you eat and drink," she explained. "You'll learn very quickly how your digestive system works and how fast your bag fills up."

"How am I going to empty it?" I asked, still trying to take it all in.

"When you sit on the toilet; position the bag between your legs, release the clip, and the contents of the bag will drain into the bowl. When you're done, take some tissue and clean the end of the bag, fold it and fasten the clip, and you're on your way."

"Okay," I replied skeptically, "but what about the smell?"

"Not a problem. The new appliances today are so good they prevent that. The only odor you will have is when you empty the pouch in the bathroom. But, that's no different from any normal person."

Melba smiled, seeming to know just what I was thinking. "Don't worry. You're going to do just fine. There may even be a day when you will actually look back at all of this and count your blessings. Life has a funny way of getting our attention and then making sure we learn what is really important."

Making a Comeback

I'm not going to sugarcoat what happened over the next month in the hospital. Complications set in, and I almost needed a third surgery. I was exhausted and depressed. I hated the constant blood draws, the changing of my IVs and dressings, and the many ways I lost my dignity. The morphine and other painkillers caused hallucinations and made sleep difficult.

But I also experienced God's mercy and the love of my family and friends. I learned to live moment-by-moment and what it took to get through each day. I tried not to worry about the future and, instead, focused on my little "victories." It was a milestone when I could get out of bed without assistance, walk three trips down the hall instead of two, and blow my breathing apparatus and finally make the ball go all the way to the top five times in a row.

When it came time to be discharged, my doctors decided that I should spend the first few weeks recuperating at my parent's house. Upon arrival, I weighed myself on the family scale. I was one hundred and twenty-six pounds, almost sixty pounds below what I was listed at in the Chargers' media guide!

I turned to my mother and smirked, "My new playing weight."

What wasn't so amusing was learning to change my appliances for the first time without Melba's help. The prospect frightened me.

The day finally came. Mom and I carefully arranged all of the supplies in front of us and began the procedure by cutting the faceplates. No sooner had we removed one of the worn-out appliances when the stoma began to ooze. Caught unprepared, all we could do was watch in horror as the waste matter leaked onto my stomach and slid slowly onto my clothes. Of course, the foul smell was not pleasant for either of us.

We quickly wiped up and continued.

"We've got to clean the skin around the stoma before we apply the adhesive paste," Mom reminded me. Sensing some urgency, Mom began to help me with the skin prep, but as if on cue, the stoma began to ooze again. In the fumbling for a towel, Mom managed to drop the paste container on the floor and knock over a glass of water next to me on the table.

"Not again!" Mom said in a frustrated voice.

We were living Murphy's Law: Anything that could go wrong did go wrong. We made four or five attempts at cleaning around the stoma, prepping the skin, and applying the paste before we were finally able to position the stupid bag. A procedure that should have taken no longer than the time it takes to kick a game-winning field goal took us forty-five agonizing minutes.

"This is ridiculous," I declared in anger. "Is the rest of my life going to be like this?"

It would take several more stabs at changing my appliances to get the hang of them, weeks to get back on my feet, and months to heal. As I slowly began to regain my strength and learn to live with the appliances, I began to wonder secretly if I could possibly kick again. Without telling anyone except the Charger's conditioning coach, I became a man on a mission and set my sights on the opening of training camp in July.

If I successfully regained my position on the team, I would become the first NFL player to compete while wearing an ostomy appliance, but that prospect seemed like light years away. First, I had to convince the doctors and myself that I could properly protect the stomas and convince the skeptics that I could kick again.

I don't think my coaches held out much hope when training camp finally rolled around that summer, but I had worked really hard to get back into shape and kicked well. I think what finally sealed the deal and helped me win my job back was kicking a 55-yarder in our third preseason game. It would be the longest kick in my career and convinced my coaches that I was back at full strength.

I ended up playing seven more seasons in the NFL, experiencing some great moments along the way. I was named Comeback Player of the Year in 1980, earned a spot in the Pro Bowl in 1982, and was named the NFL "Man of the Year" in 1983. My career highlight was kicking the game-winning field goal against the Miami Dolphins in a 1982 playoff game that *Sports Illustrated* would later call the second greatest game in NFL history.

My football career was a lot of fun, but when I got sick with ulcerative colitis, I was forced to learn that there was more to life than Sunday afternoon football games. I learned that while life is not always fair, we have a choice: we can fold out of the game, or we can play the hand we have been dealt and hope that the next hand is better. I feel so fortunate that so many people encouraged me to keep at it, people who convinced me that life is always worth fighting for, no matter how difficult it may seem at the time.

I am now married to an incredible wife, Mary, and we have four very special children. Our lives are rich beyond measure, and I realize that God has gifted me with a second chance at life, just like the individuals you'll meet in the stories that follow. I hope these people inspire you to not only survive whatever it is you are going through, but to really fight to return to *Embracing Life* and doing the things that you are really passionate about.

Good luck, and know that you are not alone.

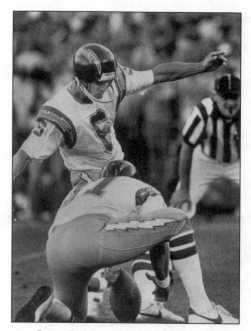
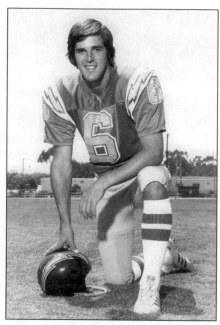

I was the second-to-last player taken in the 1977 NFL draft, and was fortunate to end up playing in my hometown for the San Diego Chargers. I would surprise everyone, including myself, by playing ten seasons, setting 16 team records, and retiring as the third-most accurate kicker in NFL history.

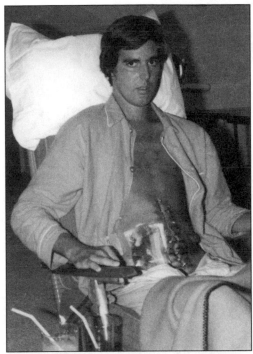

I went from kicking field goals for the San Diego Chargers on Sundays to wondering if life was worth living following my ostomy surgery in 1979. Wire sutures held my surgical incision together.

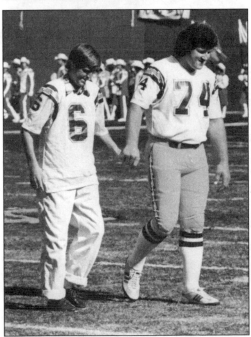

A short time after being released from the hospital in 1979 and barely strong enough to walk, the team invited me back to the stadium to watch an important match-up with the Pittsburgh Steelers. Just prior to the game, the players named me honorary captain for the day, which required me to participate in the pre-game coin-toss. The spontaneous encouragement I received from the Charger fans that day, and the support from Louie Kelcher and other teammates, would play a vital role in my recovery and provide much of the inspiration I needed to come back and play again.

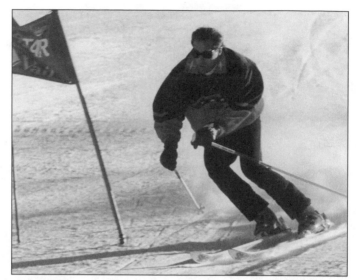

Ostomy surgery hasn't stopped me from participating in the sports that I love, including skiing, biking, scuba diving, tennis, and golf.

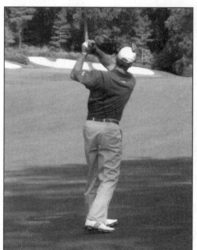

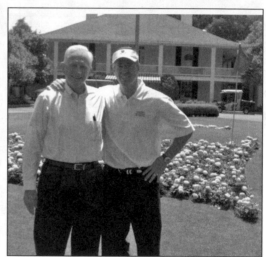

I've even had the privilege of playing Augusta National with legendary Arkansas football coach, Frank Broyles, where we made some fantastic memories.

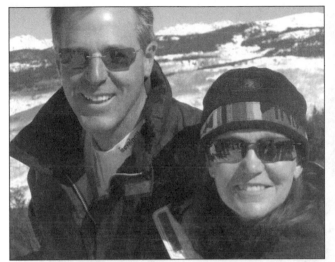

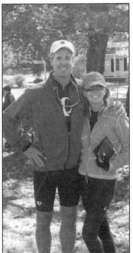

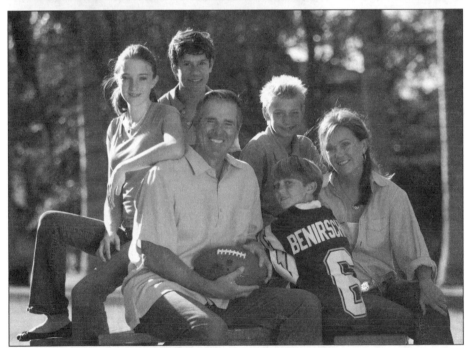

My family means everything to me, and I don't know where I'd be today without the love of my life, Mary. We've been married close to twenty years now and are in the midst of the exciting teen years with Kari, Erik (seated next to each other), and Tim. Ryan (in my old Charger jersey) will soon join them.

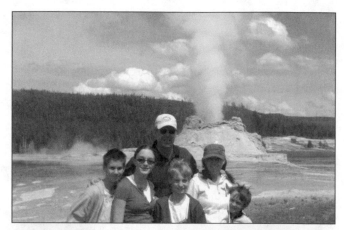

We love to travel as a family and have enjoyed Yellowstone National Park and Lake Tahoe.

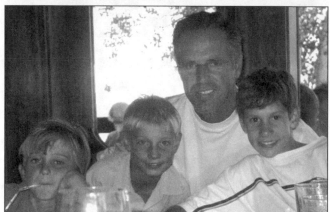

Kari loves her companion dog, Cinders, who has really become part of the family.

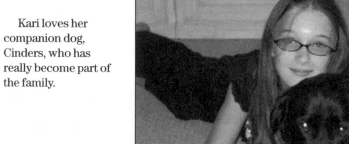

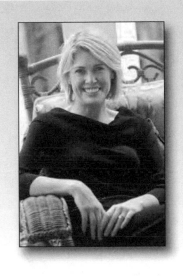

Lisa Becker

AGE: 31

HOMETOWN: Tampa, Florida

MEDICAL SITUATION:
A young woman's life takes an unexpected turn as she battles Crohn's disease that leads to an ostomy—and a new career designing and marketing special underwear for ostomy patients.

L isa Becker's story may put a new spin on the old adage, "When life hands you lemons, make lemonade." As applied to Lisa, the maxim might go something like this: "When life hands you poor health, make ... *underwear?*"

Okay, so maybe this saying lacks the panache of the former axiom, but this seemingly insignificant garment—the lowly undergarment beneath clothes—is the end result of Lisa's unglamorous fight with Crohn's disease, a battle that culminated in a nightmarish six-week hospital stay she barely survived.

Although Lisa spent most of her teens and twenties dealing with stomach ailments ranging from irritating to invasive, doctors didn't really get involved until she was around twelve years old. It would still take them another two years to figure out she was dealing with Crohn's disease. Lisa coped reasonably well throughout high school and college, relying primarily on a close network of friends who rallied to her cause whenever she had any sort of a crisis. Her worst flare-ups seemed to occur during times of stress, like a particularly difficult time near the end of her senior year of college.

A finance major at the University of Scranton in northeast Pennsylvania, Lisa managed to avoid a full-blown health crisis until the fall semester of her senior year, a time when most business majors interview for jobs. "It was an extremely competitive environment," said the thirty-one-year-old former financial analyst, who was one of only four women on campus majoring in finance. "I remember dropping off our résumés at these prominent firms in New York City hoping some one would notice us. Out of about five hundred resumes, I was one of twenty-eight who actually secured a campus interview and one of only four who were selected to go to New York for a final round of interviews. And I was the *only* person from the University of Scranton business school to actually get an offer from Goldman Sachs."

Landing such a prestigious job was more than a mere status symbol for the twenty-one-year-old, who already knew she would need a career with a decent salary and benefits in order to finance her burgeoning medical expenses.

"When November came and I got the offer, I was really psyched, but the whole process must have taken a toll on me because by December 1998, I was in a full-fledged flare-up. I ended up being hospitalized for about ten days. When I was finally discharged, my doctor advised me to take a semester off. But I had just gotten my dream job! There was no way I could put off graduating. I called all my professors and explained what was going on, and they agreed to let me do my work from home. Then I talked my roommates into shuffling my books and papers back and forth to school for a couple of weeks. I kept up with my coursework from my bed until I got strong enough to return to classes, and somehow I was able to graduate on time."

The summer after graduation Lisa found an apartment in Hoboken, New Jersey, and by July 1999 she was commuting back and forth into Manhattan, where she was starting her career in finance doing "grunt work," as she put it.

"I remember the hours being torturous. By the end of that year, right around the holidays, I got sick again. Fortunately, the company let me hop around to different departments. In October 2000, I transferred to Tampa, Florida, where I worked as a financial analyst in Goldman's Investment Management Division." It was in Tampa she began dating Stephen Becker, one of the co-workers she'd trained with at Goldman, who came frequently to Tampa on business.

She knew almost immediately that he was the one when he volunteered to drive her to a colonoscopy appointment. "I guess I reacted badly to the anesthesia because when I woke up, I got sick; Steve actually held the bedpan for me while I threw up. I remember looking up at him and saying, 'Technically, this is our second date, and you're holding a bedpan under my mouth. I must be marrying you.'"

Wedding Bells

Their path to the altar was fairly quick. In 2002, Lisa resigned from Goldman Sachs and entered the MBA program at the University of Tampa. She finished the two-year program in a year, and a few months later she and Steve were married. To their delight and surprise, Lisa conceived within a year. A daughter, Anna Victoria Becker, was born in July 2005, and, in a sense, it's here that Lisa's story really begins.

"All my life I had been told I would probably have difficulty getting pregnant," said Lisa, explaining why the newlyweds didn't even bother using protection. "Then, when I did conceive, I actually felt the best I've ever felt in my entire life. I guess the hormones acted like a natural steroid. I didn't know, however, that women with Crohn's disease have a very high chance of getting really sick *after* childbirth. If I'd taken the appropriate precautions, maybe I wouldn't have gotten as sick as I did. I now better understand the toll that pregnancy and breastfeeding take on a woman's body, but at the time, I was on an adrenaline high that lasted several months after Anna's birth."

Needless to say, after the rush wore off, Lisa's system went haywire, and nothing she did to manage this latest flare-up worked. In the past, she could usually bring things under control by either staying in bed all day, or by putting herself on a liquid diet, or as a last resort, by involving her doctor. But that was before Anna entered the picture.

"Anna became the X-factor. I didn't have the luxury of sleeping all day or manipulating my diet. And even though Steve came to my aid more than he ever had before, nothing helped, not even drugs. When you've had Crohn's disease for a long time, you get to know your body, and in the back of my mind, I knew this flare-up was different from all the others—it was too severe, too deep."

As the year progressed, it became increasingly difficult for Lisa to cope, especially after the baby became more mobile and she was forced to spend more time in the bathroom. "Sometimes I'd put her in the bathtub next to me while I was on the toilet so I could keep an eye on her. I remember one time being in Target when she was about nine months old and bringing her into the stall. I sang nursery rhymes at the top of my lungs to distract her from the horrible sounds my body was making. When you're losing your insides as violently as I was, it's not a pretty sight . . . or sound! I remember thinking I don't want her to know me like this."

The tipping point came a short time later while Lisa was driving to the grocery store. "I remember getting the 'signal' from my body and realizing I had about ten seconds to get to a bathroom. Those ten seconds, however, didn't include unlatching my baby from her car seat and carrying her into the bathroom. I literally did not know what to do. Of course, I soiled my pants. I totally lost it. Before Anna, when I was on my own, I was always able to manage this disease, but now it was different. Now it was invading my ability to be a mother. I cried all the way home because I knew what I needed to do."

Understanding that her doctor would hospitalize her the minute she contacted him, Lisa held off making the call until after Anna's first birthday. She didn't even tell Steve about her decision because he was in the middle of an important presentation at work. Instead, she asked a friend to drive her to the appointment. When her gastroenterologist entered the office, she immediately burst into tears.

"I had done absolutely no reading about ostomy surgery, and I didn't even know what an ostomy bag looked like, but I told him I wanted the surgery . . . *needed* the surgery! He tried to talk me out of it, but I told him you don't understand how bad it's gotten. I'm *done.*"

The two went back and forth, Lisa insisting she needed surgery, and her doctor, who'd been treating her for years, suggesting they try less invasive methods first. There was a new drug called Humira that he was hearing good things about. It hadn't been approved for Crohn's patients yet, but he thought it might do the trick if Lisa's insurance policy would agree to pay for it. Ultimately, Lisa agreed to let him try the new drug therapy, but deep in her heart she was convinced it wouldn't work. Twenty-four hours later, she entered Tampa General Hospital for what she thought would be no more than a short visit.

Her hospital stay ended up being a lot longer.

An Unforgettable Case

The nurses who attended to Lisa that summer told her later she should have kept a journal of those weeks. Some people have suggested she write a book. Maybe some day she will. "The whole experience was surreal," mused Lisa as she recalled a deluge of complications and calamities that might border on the ludicrous if the outcome hadn't been so grave.

She still shakes her head when she thinks about that summer at the hospital. "About a year after I was released, I ran into one of the surgical residents who helped take care of me," recalls Lisa. "When he saw me, he said, 'Lisa Becker, you are one case I will *never* forget.' I remember thinking, 'OK, so it wasn't just me—it really was that bad." Among the mishaps was an ant infestation in her hospital room and a family member tripping over her TPN line, but those were the least consequential (though no less distressing) events she and Steve were forced to contend with.

The more serious complications—a life-threatening blood clot in her lung, deep vein thrombosis in her arms, six blood transfusions, collapsing veins, botched pain management, a massive intestinal blockage, and a potentially-fatal systemic infection—portray an escalating state of affairs that forced a young couple to make monumental decisions about issues they'd never thought to discuss until then.

Lisa's husband, Steve—who ended up taking a long leave of absence to be with Lisa during this ordeal—said virtually every day brought another round of bad news. "It was almost as if you had to distance yourself from reality and handle each problem as it arose rather than getting caught up in it all," he said. "You didn't have time to stop and think about whether she was going to live or die. We seemed to be in crisis mode all of the time . . . forced to deal with one crisis and then move on to the next."

While waiting on approval for the Humira, Lisa's doctor tried the usual protocol—IV's, steroids, bowel rest—but there was just no let-up. "I was going to the bathroom thirty to forty times a day, and each time blood would come gushing out," said Lisa, who refused to use a bedpan until the very end. Once the approval came, her doctor was confident that this drug would do the trick since he had seen it work on patients who were in worse shape than Lisa.

Indeed, from all appearances, Lisa's condition seemed to start improving. She became chipper and more positive, and even managed to look "pretty in pink" from day to day. As is often the case, though, appearances can be deceiving. Ironically, it may have been Lisa's innate optimism and spunky personality that obscured what was really going on.

"I worked very hard to look at the positive side," said Lisa, whose striking good looks and personal charisma are enhanced by a genuinely engaging smile. "I wore my own pajamas instead of a hospital gown and tied my hair back every day just to keep some semblance of normalcy. But the doctor interpreted those actions as a sign that I was on the mend, which just wasn't the case at all."

Lisa vividly remembers the day when it became clear that she was not only not mending but was actually deteriorating. "They had done a scope of my rectum when I first arrived," she explained, "but after three weeks of drug therapy, my doctor wanted to check on my progress, so he scheduled another scope. I knew I was worse and even said so. The morning when I went in for the procedure, I told my doctor and Steve not to be too disappointed when they found out how bad things really were."

Sure enough, when Lisa woke up from anesthesia, both Steve and her normally composed doctor had tears in their eyes. They informed her she would need surgery—and soon. "Everyone had had such high hopes that we could beat this," Steve admitted later. "We'd been there for three weeks, had tried everything, including Humira, which we were made to think would do the trick. Now her colon was actually *worse* than it was when we'd first arrived. We were right back to where we started."

A Turn for the Worse

Then Lisa began to experience what she thought were gas pains. Her nurses felt she might be having an anxiety attack, but when her heart rate shot up to 160 beats per minute, twice her normal resting rate, she was rushed to the lab for a CT scan. It turned out that Lisa had neither gas nor anxiety but a pulmonary embolism—a potentially life-threatening blood clot in her lung.

At the time, she didn't really know what that meant, but she guessed right away that the situation was dire. Unfortunately, it was after hours on a Sunday night in the university-affiliated teaching hospital, so her personal physician was not available. She remembers the ER doctor being "so freaked out, he didn't know what to do." When she called a friend who happened to be a doctor and told him what was happening, "He did a U-turn on a major highway and raced to the hospital."

In order to dissolve the clot, Lisa began receiving injections of an anticoagulant called Lovenox. While the treatment no doubt saved her life, the injections ultimately put her in a precarious situation. Her predicament was aptly summed up by one of the residents assigned to her case.

"You were like a sinking ship," the doctor commented in a moment of unexpected candor days later. "On one end of the ship, you had such a bad case of Crohn's disease that we needed to do surgery, but on the other end of the ship, you had a dangerous blood clot in your lung that was requiring us to keep you on blood thinners. We knew we needed to take you off blood thinners so we could do the surgery, but you needed the blood thinners to keep you alive. We were in a terrible predicament and didn't know which side of the ship we should try to fix first."

Eventually the doctors had no choice but to take her off blood thinners until they could proceed with the surgery. To protect her heart, they inserted a vena cava filter through the main jugular vein in her neck to act as a kind of screen. Emergency surgery was scheduled for a Saturday morning, but complications plagued the procedure from the outset.

Doctors discovered deep vein thrombosis—more blood clots— in her arm. To make matters worse, she had explosive diarrhea just moments before the anesthesia was administered. It was Steve that sprang into action and quickly shoved a bedpan under his wife's dressing gown just in time, startling the anesthesiologist, who seemed quite caught off guard by the unexpected disruption.

Even more disturbing to the doctor, however, was when Lisa emerged from anesthesia screaming out in pain. No amount of morphine seemed to lessen her discomfort. It would take two days before a pain management specialist discovered that her spinal anesthesia hadn't been properly inserted. "Those idiots didn't check that?" the woman questioned, clearly irritated at what Lisa was made to endure.

Then, on the day she was scheduled to be discharged, Lisa began spewing green bile "like a violent hose," she explained. It turned out she had something called an ileus, or blockage, because her digestive system had shut down from all of the anesthesia. To make a dismal situation even more dire, an abscess near the top of her rectum burst, releasing a massive amount of bacteria into her body, causing a major infection. She would end up spending another week in varying states of consciousness before finally being allowed to go home.

Did she nearly die? She's not sure. Steve says it was definitely a "serious situation." Lisa doesn't remember much, other than having an overwhelming yearning to be with Anna. "That was the hardest part of the whole experience. I was missing my little girl, and my heart was aching." She remembers thinking, *Don't let your heart break. Turn your broken heart into strength. You have to get out of here.*

The day she finally came home was "pretty emotional," but that was really just the beginning of her recovery. She had been "filleted down the middle," could hardly move without pain, and yet she refused to take anything stronger than Tylenol. Her body would take longer to heal because of the residual prednisone that had to be weaned out of her system, and she was still weak from the infection. But despite all of that, she found a way to bond again with Anna, propping her up with pillows and deeply inhaling the recognizable fragrance of her only child.

The perceptive little girl became so attuned to her mother's discomfort that within two weeks of Lisa's return, she knew exactly where the pillows were stored behind the rocking chair. When Anna wanted to cuddle, she would drag them out and place them gently on Lisa's lap before climbing up for her bottle. Rather than clamor to be picked up, she learned to tug on Lisa's hand so the two could hug on the floor.

"Children pick up on so much more than you think," explained Lisa, still clearly moved as she recalled the early adjustments they all needed to make. She added that Anna, now an energetic preschooler, wasn't completely unaffected by her mother's absence and long convalescence. She gets very anxious whenever Lisa is gone for even a short period of time and just recently developed a stammer. But Lisa is determined to use what has happened as a way to set a positive example in her daughter's life. Like all mothers, she is careful about what she exposes her daughter to, but she doesn't hide the fact that she has an ostomy.

"Having a child makes you so much more aware of how you verbalize things. When Anna asks about my stoma, I explain that Mommy had a big boo-boo, but the doctors fixed it, and now Mommy is so happy. I want her to know that even though there are obstacles in life, you can always find a way to get around them. I believe that God only gives you as much as He thinks you can handle. I know that there are so many awful things that can happen to someone, but having an ostomy isn't one of them. I believe completely that my ostomy gave me back my life, my health, and my freedom."

Fashion Statement

Which brings us back to underwear. As soon as Lisa got used to life with an ostomy, she realized how much she *despised* those oversized shirts and bulky clothes she had been wearing to conceal her ostomy bag. She wasn't crazy about palazzo pants and skirts. She wanted to get back into the clothes she was accustomed to wearing—like low-cut jeans and sexy tanks. She wanted to look *cute* again. But there was one problem: the ostomy bag hanging from her belly didn't exactly make her feel cute and sexy but rather self-conscious and unattractive. She decided to do something about it.

"A few months after I got home, I became obsessed about wanting to wear my old clothes again. It started with sleepless nights where I spent hours researching ostomies on the Internet. I went on message boards and read what people had to say, and what I read completely freaked me out. You won't believe the extremes some people go to. I heard about people literally taping the bag to their legs so they could wear their own clothes. I read about a woman my age who refused to leave the house and wouldn't tell anyone what had happened to her. I discovered that some people get divorced after ostomy surgery because they're so ashamed of themselves.

"I learned people are terrified of this surgery. They're afraid of what they're going to look like or what people might think of them. They wonder if they'll ever feel attractive again or if they'll ever be able to enjoy sex again with their spouses. I understood their fears. When you have an ostomy, the one thing you do lose is your body image. No wonder—a bag of excrement dangling from one's abdomen is certainly a deterrent to a positive self-image."

The idea of self-image really consumed Lisa. The more she researched, the more she became convinced that if people could somehow forget they had an ostomy bag attached to their bodies, the better they would feel about themselves. Intuitively, she knew that this was the job of underwear. What was needed was a garment worn beneath the clothing that would support the ostomy bag and keep it from bulging as it filled. It made perfect sense, and that's how her obsession began.

At first, she experimented with different styles of panties that she purchased from department stores. She even bought a sewing machine so she could try her hand at design, even though she admits she's not a seamstress. When that approach failed, she went online and discovered companies outside the United States that marketed underwear for people with ostomies. She ordered samples and tried them on. The results were dramatic.

"It's amazing how something as seemingly insignificant as underwear can make a difference," said Lisa with a smile. "I remember thinking that I would pay $100 for this garment just because it was worth that much to me for the way it made me feel. And then I thought, *Everybody who has an ostomy needs this underwear.*" The seed of an idea was born.

The garments Lisa had ordered from the United Kingdom weren't what you'd call *pretty.* "They were more medical garb than underwear," she recalled, "but how hard would it be to design underwear for men and women that were both functional *and* attractive?"

In December 2007, Lisa shared her ideas with a family friend, Christina Ebner, who came for a visit during the Christmas holidays. "I brought her up to my bathroom and showed her all the underwear I had ordered," said Lisa. "I even modeled for her so she could see how they worked. There I stood, full-blown naked in front of her, explaining that women with ostomies *need* this underwear, and men needed their own ostomy underwear as well. Christina just looked at me with a big grin and said, 'I can totally help you with this. I'm in the design industry. This is what I *do!*'"

And that's how their company, Ostomy Secrets, was born. The two women began searching for manufacturers to help produce their new line of underwear. Steve and Lisa plunked down their savings ("I have the most amazing husband") to fund the effort, and Christina began designing the products that would not only include traditional panties for women and boxers for men, but also "peek-a-boo" thongs and sexy "vixen wraps" for those intimate moments. Christina also creates all the spec packages for the manufacturers and helps Lisa with marketing. They plan to begin selling Ostomy Secrets products online in 2009. (Go to www.ostomysecrets.com for more information about ordering your own "special" underwear.)

For Lisa, who admits she's "wired naturally" to focus on money, explains that this venture is not about getting rich. Indeed, she's well aware that today's uncertain economic climate is probably not the best time to be starting a business. If she doesn't make a dime, however, she wouldn't care. "Ostomy Secrets is my passion," she said, pointing out that there isn't a huge profit margin for selling underwear anyway.

"All I care about is seeing what happens to the faces of patients. I was in the hospital just a couple of days ago visiting a twenty-nine-year-old cancer patient who had a temporary ileostomy. He was absolutely devastated. I showed him a couple of our prototypes, and he literally cried. He thanked me and said, 'You don't know how much this means to me.' I just looked at him and said, 'You're wrong—I know *exactly* how much this means to you.'

"For me that's what this is all about. It's about feeling good about you again. As crazy as it sounds, I really believe everything I've been through in my life—including having this ostomy—comes down to this. Ostomy Secrets is my mission. This is what I'm supposed to be doing."

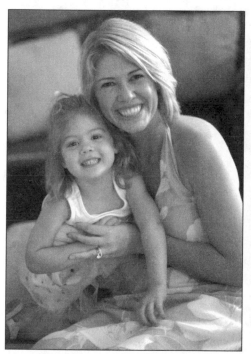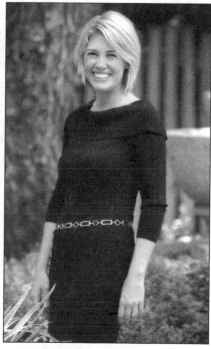

Lisa Becker told her three-year-old daughter, Anna, that she had a big "boo-boo" but the doctors fixed it, and now Mommy's happy. Lisa now designs functional and attractive underwear for ostomates called Ostomy Secrets. (Visit www.ostomysecrets.com for more information.)

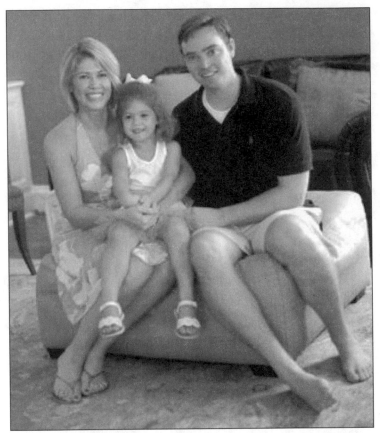

Lisa isn't sure how she would have made it without the incredible support of her husband, Steve, but today she appreciates her health and her little girl, Anna, more than ever.

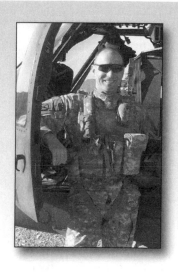

Robert Cuyler

AGE: 43

HOMETOWN: Hannibal, New York

MEDICAL SITUATION:
A U.S. Army helicopter pilot, grounded by severe ulcerative colitis, submits to ileostomy surgery that should end his military career . . .

You would think that being deployed to Afghanistan and battling the Taliban and Al Qaeda would be enough for any soldier, but Chief Warrant Officer Robert Cuyler, a U.S. Army helicopter pilot, found himself fighting a two-front war: one against terrorism and the other against ulcerative colitis.

The bad guys he could handle; it was the inflammatory bowel disease that took no prisoners. For months in Afghanistan, he endured painful digestive episodes that compromised his ability to serve and to live a normal life, but he never complained. Toward the end of his second tour, his body was racked by an intense flare-up, and this time around, Bob had to accept a battlefield retreat. He was medically evacuated to Germany and eventually the United States to recover from his wounds, but constant bleeding led to anemia and a loss of appetite.

Two months after leaving the Afghan war theater, his military-lean body had shed fifty pounds. When a colonoscopy revealed that his colon was over 85 percent diseased, his superiors told him his military career was over and he'd never fly again.

At this point, Bob had been fighting ulcerative colitis for seven years, and while he held his ground during that time, the enemy continued to advance. Finally, in the summer of 2007, Bob and his wife, Tammy, had to admit defeat. He waved the white flag of surrender and submitted to a total proctocolectomy, which meant the removal of his entire colon, leaving him with an ileostomy.

After a month of convalescent leave, Bob was told to report to the Warrior Transition Unit (WTU), which could mean only one thing: the U.S. Army no longer had use for a helicopter pilot with an ostomy bag attached to his abdomen. The WTU caseworker informed Bob that the military had decided to start the "separation process," a military euphemism for getting the discharge paperwork going.

After completing numerous medical forms and questionnaires, Bob met with a young doctor who immediately began explaining the Army's medical evaluation and separation process. During the middle of his memorized routine, he stopped—as if he could sense that Bob wasn't ready to give up his military career. He then explained how the Army would calculate the physical disability compensation, which was clearly based on capabilities and limitations.

"How can the Army determine this if we don't know what my capabilities or limitations are?" Bob asked, even though he was still very weak.

"Well, you have an ostomy," replied the doctor matter-of-factly.

"Is there any possibility of staying on active duty by being a classroom instructor at the schoolhouse?" Bob pressed.

The doctor thought for a moment before responding. "We have two choices here," he said. "We can do the paperwork now, and you'll be out of the Army in a matter of weeks, or, if you would like, we could slow the process down a bit and see what happens. It's entirely up to you. As for staying on active duty, a medical evaluation board will have to decide if your condition doesn't pose a problem in a stateside assignment. Maybe then they would let you stay in."

Bob, scared at the prospects of losing his military career and leaving what he loved to do, understood that the system was in motion to discharge him. The regular route would be taking the medical separation and turning to the next chapter in his life.

But then Bob kept recalling stories that he had just read in a book, *Great Comebacks from Ostomy Surgery*, given to him by his ostomy nurse. He was amazed at what the people in the book were able to accomplish after their ostomy surgery, like returning to their careers as a firefighter or ski film cinematographer. One fellow, Dave Alberga, even competed in mini-triathlons just months after his ostomy surgery.

Bob knew he was at a major crossroads in his life—a point where the main road headed straight with all the signs saying "Easy Out," but off to the side was a tiny sign pointing into the dark that said, "Military Career."

Should he just accept a medical separation and take the benefits being offered to him? Or should Bob follow an untraveled path to see if there was something the Army might be willing to let him do?

It was a decision that had been building his entire life.

Pitching In at an Early Age

Bob Cuyler's story begins in the small upstate New York town of Hannibal, where he was the fourth of six children born to Lavern and Lois Cuyler. Their family lived on a small farm, and when the children were old enough, everyone was expected to pitch in with the farm chores to keep things going. Beginning in elementary school, Bob picked beans and peas, and his nimble fingers plucked ripe tomatoes from the vine. There wasn't much time for organized sports when fall came around since his father needed help cutting down trees for the family's side business—selling firewood.

When he was in seventh grade, his parents informed him that

he was now expected to purchase all of his own school clothes. "I got my working papers at thirteen so I could pick strawberries that summer," Bob recalled. "I remember being so excited to earn money and buy my own things. I didn't think it was a big deal to buy my own school clothes. That's what my older brother and sisters all had to do."

Despite having to work on weekends and during the summer, Bob managed to play football and baseball throughout high school. During his senior year, Bob decided he wanted to go to college. That would be fine, his father replied, but he needed to find a way to pay for his schooling. As Bob looked at his options, joining the Air National Guard looked appealing since that qualified him to have his college bills partially paid for in exchange for a six-year commitment to the Air National Guard after he earned his degree.

At the age of seventeen, and still in high school, Bob joined the Air National Guard. Immediately following graduation, he attended Air Force Basic Training at Lackland Air Force Base outside of San Antonio, Texas, followed by Engineering Assistant Technical School at nearby Shepard Air Force Base.

After his military training in Texas, Bob returned to New York to attend State University of New York (SUNY) at Morrisville. He married his high school sweetheart, Tammy, following graduation and took a job as a land surveyor, which had been a summertime job during his college years. Although he was just twenty-one when he married, Bob felt he and his wife were heading in the right direction—except for the times his stomach felt funny. That's when he'd have to find a bathroom in a hurry. Being young and feeling invincible, he just chalked up those every-now-and-then episodes to something he ate.

Needing work, Bob joined a professional land surveying company full time, and for the next six years, he helped buyers and sellers of property determine the dimensions of the land they were purchasing. At the age of twenty-seven, with a four-year-old daughter, Megan, and a one-year-old son, Jared, having joined the family, Bob began looking around and considering other options. Should he start his own land surveying business? Could he earn enough to support his family? Would a career in land surveying fulfill him? Is this what he wanted to do with the rest of his life?

When he was really honest with himself, the answer to the last two questions was definitely no.

It was his military service with the Air National Guard, where he served one weekend a month along with two- to four-week deployments each year, that whetted his appetite and caused him to consider a military career. He had traveled around the U.S., Europe, and Panama, working on construction projects for the U.S. military, and it was in a remote area of Panama—shortly after General Manuel Noriega's regime was overthrown in 1989—that he got his first ride in a military helicopter.

Afterward, his supervisor told him that by the look in Bob's eyes, he knew that someday he would be a helicopter pilot. Bob agreed that he had always had a secret ambition to fly an army chopper. That desire had been planted years earlier when he was eight years old and a neighbor's friend offered the wide-eyed boy the opportunity to climb into his helicopter and go for a ride. "It was a thrill I never forgot," he said.

One day while working for the land surveying company, Bob stopped at the local post office to check the mail. While there, he noticed an advertisement looking for Army aviation helicopter pilots. After reading the ad, he convinced himself that he didn't want to go through life saying to himself, "I wish I had done this when I had the chance . . . ."

Several weeks passed. Then one night after work, Bob handed Tammy a copy of the ad. "What do you think, Hon?" he said. "You know I've always wanted to fly helicopters."

Tammy knew that her husband was fast approaching twenty-seven, the cut-off age to apply to the military, and that he would always regret not giving active duty military service a chance. They both agreed that it would be a great experience for the family to travel and live in different places around the world. That evening, she gave her blessing.

The U.S. Army accepted Bob's application for the Warrant Officer Flight Training Program, and he was soon shipped to Fort Jackson in Columbia, South Carolina, for eight weeks of boot camp, followed by a six-week Warrant Officer Candidate School, followed by another year in the Warrant Officer Flight Training program at Fort Rucker near Dothan, Alabama.

Toward the end of Flight Training, his class of soon-to-be-pilots was handed a piece of paper, and they were asked to write down their preferred assignment requests. This was in 1994, three years after U.S. Army helicopters had destroyed Saddam Hussein's vaunted Republican Guard in the Iraqi desert. Although the Gulf War was over, Army helo pilots were enforcing a "no fly" zone in northern Iraq, which was considered hazardous duty. Another hot spot everyone was crossing off their list was South Korea because of the belligerence of the North Koreans, who liked to target helicopter patrols that veered too closely to North Korean airspace.

Would it be Iraq or South Korea?

This time around, Bob was assigned a one-year tour of duty in South Korea, and although he had to posted away from his family for a year, he was excited about the opportunity to progress as a pilot. Patrols along the North Korea border were like real-time "war games." The Great Leader, Kim Jong-Il, ruled the Hermit Kingdom with an iron fist and was pushing the country to produce nuclear weapons, which further raised diplomatic tensions between Pyongyang and Washington, D.C.

It didn't help matters that during Bob's tour, Army helicopter pilot Bobby Hall strayed into North Korea by mistake—a navigational error, he said, but which was viewed as a spy mission by Pyongyang.

North Korean gunfire downed Hall's OH-58A helicopter, killing Hall's co-pilot and leading to Bobby Hall's capture. It would be thirteen long, anxious days before Hall was released following a coerced confession. "We did not know if another war was going to start because of what happened to Bobby Hall," Bob recalled. "It was a very tense time for all of us, and especially harrowing for me because as part of the 2nd Infantry Division and the front line of defense against South Korea, I was flying along the border right where Bobby's chopper went down."

Thankfully, Bob's tour in South Korea passed without incident, although it was tough not seeing his family for an entire year. The only bright spot was that he could focus on improving his piloting skills.

When his tour was over, the Army gave Bob a new assignment, this time to the 10th Mountain Division at Fort Drum, New York—less than a hundred miles from their home town, Hannibal, where his family had been living while he was stationed in Korea. It was an easy move to Fort Drum for the family, who was happy to finally rejoin him and live on the base in post housing.

Surrounded by his family, loving his job, Bob was now twenty-nine years old and living the full military life. The only dark cloud was managing the occasional digestive flare-up he experienced when he was flying a helicopter, which wasn't equipped with a toilet. Fortunately, most helo flights were shorter than two hours, although sometimes training flights lasted much longer. (On those occasions, pilots could relieve themselves during refueling stops.) "Lots of times, the pressure got so bad that the only thing that mattered most was making it to a bathroom," Bob recalled. "That was pretty rough, but I'm thankful I never had an accident and soiled by pants, although they were certainly challenging times."

After three-and-a-half years at Fort Drum, Bob was reassigned again, this time to the 1st Infantry Division and stationed in Ansbach, Germany, where he was called into his first imminent danger zone—Kosovo. He was part of the first aircrew stationed in Kosovo at a military facility known as Camp Bondsteel.

"We were living in tents with portable potties, and that's where I first noticed indications of bleeding," Bob said. "The bleeding alarmed me, and I was duty bound to report to my flight surgeon what was happening. He checked me over and figured that I probably had fissures. 'Take lots of fiber,' he told me. 'Make sure you get some Metamucil.' "

Bob took that as an order, and Metamucil and orange juice became his breakfast drink of choice. His health situation didn't worsen, but it didn't improve either. Over the next several months, the frequency of bowel movements went from once or twice a day to four or five times daily. Again, he reported what was happening to his flight surgeon, who didn't show any sort of concern or worry. "You're young and healthy. Just be sure you continue to take your Metamucil," the flight surgeon instructed.

While in Germany, Bob was required to report back to Fort Rucker to take an advanced officer training course—not related to flying but to his professional development. It was supposed to be a two-month course, temporary duty, so his family stayed back in Germany while Bob traveled stateside.

Halfway through the course, he got a break and a chance to fly back to Germany to rejoin his family for Christmas. Unfortunately, the minute his holiday break was over and he stepped on board the flight back to the States in January 2001, the worst abdominal pain he had ever experienced grabbed him by the throat.

"I had the hardest time on the long transatlantic flight," Bob recalled. "When I arrived at Atlanta, I rented a car for the drive to my hotel on Fort Rucker. I remember stopping at every bathroom along the way. When I finally got to the hotel, I was bleeding continuously and fighting nausea. I immediately checked into the Fort Rucker medical clinic, and the next day I had a colonoscopy that determined I was suffering from a severe case of ulcerative colitis. When I first heard the news, I immediately began to worry about what this might mean for my career."

Doctors put Bob on 60 milligrams of prednisone right away—his first experience with the drug. "If I had a garage that needed straightening up, I could have cleaned it out ten times a day from the boost prednisone gave me," Bob recalled with a wry smile.

Meanwhile, he was medically grounded, which gave Bob time to do some poking around on the Internet and try to understand what his newly diagnosed condition was all about. That's when he found out that the U.S. Army graded ulcerative colitis as a "disqualifying condition." Unless he could get his disease into remission and show that his colon was not affected more than 25 centimeters deep, Bob would be medically discharged from the military. Bob's most recent colonoscopy showed that his ulcerative colitis was right up to the limit—25 centimeters.

Still very concerned, Bob returned to Germany and continued his prednisone treatment. Several months later, another colonoscopy was scheduled to see if the treatments were working and if it could be determined that he was in remission. Right from the beginning of the procedure, something didn't seem right. He clenched his teeth trying to endure the pain, but then he overheard the military doctor bragging to others in the operating bay that he "got all the way to the other end" by hardly using any sedatives or anesthesia with the patient.

"The first part of the colonoscopy was no problem," Bob recalled, "but I'll never forget after he had to make the bend from the ascending colon to the transverse colon. Every time he moved the colonoscope further along, it was brutally painful. He really should have had me on some kind of anesthesia."

Good news, though. The doctor said that he was in remission and recommended a temporary return to flight status while they waited for approval of a permanent medical waiver. Excited once again, Bob immediately returned to the flight line to continue his duties as an instructor pilot.

The Quest to Continue Flying

Unfortunately, bad news arrived in January 2002: Bob's request for a permanent waiver was declined because of his ulcerative colitis, even though medically speaking he was in remission. Not willing to give up without a fight, this started a year-long tug-of-war with the Army. Bob, believing he was fit and could still fly, sought medical proof that he was, in fact, in remission from ulcerative colitis, while the Army continued to try to show him the door. Because of his persistence, and with help from commanders and doctors who believed in him and really cared, Bob was granted a waiver to continue flying.

This is where he hoped his story would end. As many people with ulcerative colitis know, however, the condition rarely stays away forever. For Bob, his first new flare-up happened during his first tour in Afghanistan when he was sent over as part of Operation Enduring Freedom following the terrorist attacks of September 11th. Bob had been working out, running steadily, and lifting weights when his energy level suddenly sunk like a helo without power.

The next thing he knew, Bob was being half-carried into a medical tent, nearly delirious from weakness and fluid loss. An IV was inserted into his arm—an IV that hadn't been warmed up at all. The cold IV fluid suddenly rushing into his veins felt like an ice water bath, and Bob got a major case of the chills. "The doctor wanted to immediately evacuate me back to the States, but being as stubborn I was, I insisted on getting more prednisone so I could get this thing back into remission," Bob remembers, shaking his head. "I knew what the disease was and I knew how prednisone had worked in the past for me."

After agreeing to let Bob stay, his commander joked that he wouldn't dare send him home to his wife looking like he had just gotten out of a concentration camp. Somehow, Bob managed to recover from the flare-up and was able to finish his tour successfully.

Following a short break back in the States, Bob returned to Afghanistan in support of Operation Enduring Freedom. He was back up in the air and seemed to be healthy again. "I was working out every day and could score the maximum amount on the Army's physical fitness test," Bob recalled. But then, unexplainable pain and swelling in all his major joints—elbows, wrists, shoulder, knees, and ankles—appeared and began taking their toll.

By the end of his second tour, he was on crutches and hurt all over. Bloody diarrhea became his constant companion, and this time he had to be medically evacuated. Weight fell off like he had dropped his combat body armor to the floor. From a buff 190 pounds, Bob's weight dipped to 140 pounds—and with it all of his energy.

He was told that there wasn't much else that could be done except to keep taking high doses of prednisone. The common side effects—irritability and shortness with others—began presenting themselves. Although Bob knew what to expect, he found himself snapping at Tammy or losing his patience with the kids. "No matter how hard I tried to be patient and not get irritated, I still was," Bob said with resignation in his voice.

Yet Bob was willing to keep trying the high doses of prednisone because he wanted desperately to try to keep from having ostomy surgery. He knew that once his colon was removed, it would be the end of his military career, *finito*. His days of flying a helicopter would be over.

"I didn't know the difference between a colostomy and an ileostomy," Bob said. "All I knew was that they both involved having a bag, and I didn't want that."

By now, Bob had learned that his colon was 85 percent diseased. One doctor informed him on a scale of 1-10, with 10 being the best, his health was a 1.4. Bob didn't disagree with him and realized he was out of options. The time had come to submit to a colectomy.

Then the Army threw him a curve. The chain of command informed him that they were going to officially turn him over to the Veteran's health care system for treatment and surgery. "Now, it's hard to say something without insulting people," Bob explained, "but I told them I didn't want to have a total colectomy done at the

Veteran's Hospital. I was very comfortable with the physicians who were now treating me." Because soldiers and doctors are constantly moving, continuity of care is not the norm in the military.

While there was no way he could remain in the Army after his total colectomy, he did win the battle to have the procedure done by the surgeons that he was comfortable with. This action lifted his spirits, and on July 27, 2007, Bob had his total proctocolectomy done.

During his recovery in the hospital, he was surprised one day when his nurse dropped by with a present. "You really need to read this book," she said, handing him a copy of *Great Comebacks from Ostomy Surgery*. Intrigued, Bob devoured its contents, and couldn't stop thinking about the inspirational people the book profiled. Each had undergone ostomy surgery, and each had not only rebuilt their lives but returned to doing the things that they were most passionate about. Many resumed engaging in amazing physical activities.

It was about that time when Bob was told to report to the WTU—the Warrior Transition Unit. Buoyed by the stories he had just read, Bob stalled for time by suggesting to his superiors that surely there was *something* he could do in the Army—perhaps be an instructor pilot or teach in the classroom. His persistence won him several delays, which he used to work on getting back his physical conditioning. Every morning at 0700, Bob was pumping iron in the gym, going out on four-mile runs, and marching double time with an oversized backpack across his back.

His commanders noticed, and several began to wonder if he really was "disabled." As if to see how he would do, he was allowed to join his unit on a month-long combat training exercise in Fort Polk, Louisiana, where everyone lived in a combat environment under austere conditions in hot and humid weather. Bob not only kept up physically, he performed well in the exercises—so well that a flight surgeon, who had been watching his recovery closely and secretly pulling for him, one day handed him an up-slip to fly. "If you stand a chance of getting approval from the Army to ever fly again, we have to get you in the cockpit to show that you have no limitations," he said.

Bob Cuyler was overjoyed and knew he was close to being back to where he belonged. He was sure of it. The only thing left to do now was to convince a military board that he could return to full active duty as a helicopter pilot.

Bob remembers the day vividly when a ten-person board, made up of seven doctors and three pilots, deliberated nearly ninety minutes over what to do. They held Bob's flying future in their hands as they weighed all of the evidence to determine whether he would be able to carry out all of his responsibilities as a pilot and if he could be relied upon in the most severe of combat circumstances.

When the door finally opened and he was informed that the Army board had indeed granted him a permanent waiver to continue flying, even in a combat zone, Bob could hardly believe the great news. He had waited outside that chamber fretting and wondering if all that he had gone through was worth it.

"I will never forget the feeling," Bob said, visibly moved. "It was as if somebody took my career and handed it back to me."

Serving Our Country

In October 2008, Bob was rewarded for his persistence and hard work when he was deployed to Iraq for a twelve-month tour as a helicopter pilot. All the research he has done shows that he is the first U.S. soldier to be deployed with an ostomy *and* the first Army aviator to fly in a combat zone with an ostomy.

"My worries aren't about flying or combat or of what I'll find there, but of what I leave behind," Bob said upon his departure. "My wife, Tammy, my daughter, Megan, and my son, Jared, have all been there for me every step of the way. They have sacrificed so much through the military years. The last time I deployed, Megan was a senior in high school, and I missed her graduation. Jared is a senior this time. My wife does so much when I'm home, but she does everything when I'm gone. Please put them in your prayers."

Bob knew his family had been looking forward to the possibility of him getting out of the military and being around all of the time. But they also saw how important serving his country and flying was to him, and they continue to support him in every way.

The bottom line for Bob Cuyler is that after rigorous physical conditioning and intense scrutiny by medical physicians, his commanders feel that he posed no risk to himself or anybody else when serving his country in the fight against terrorism.

And that's something we can all be thankful for.

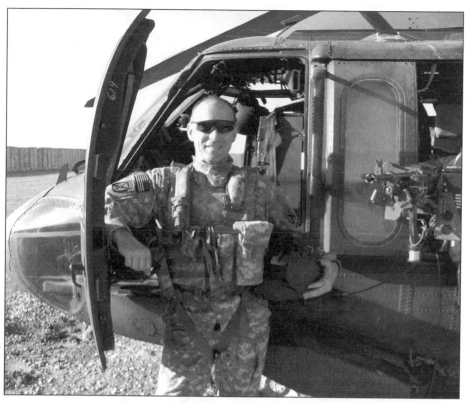

U.S. Army helicopter pilot Robert Cuyler has two remarkable credits to his career: he's the first U.S. soldier to be deployed with an ostomy and the first Army aviator to fly in a combat zone with an ostomy.

Embrace LIFE

HABÍA UNA VEZ . . . OR ONCE UPON A TIME

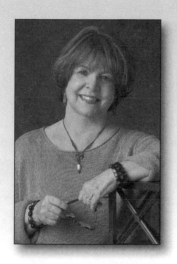

Sandra Benitez

AGE: 67

HOMETOWN: Edina, Minnesota

MEDICAL SITUATION:
A young American girl growing up
in El Salvador begins experiencing
ulcerative colitis at the age of five and
suffers in silence for nearly fifty years . . .
until she undergoes life-changing
ileostomy surgery.

In her recently published memoir, *bag lady: A Memoir*, Sandra Benitez tells about a time years ago when she purchased an old flat-topped trunk from an antique store in St. Louis. The trunk was locked, it was heavy, and there was no key. Something was inside—but what?

Many people dream of discovering lost secrets and hidden wealth in locked trunks, and Sandra was no exception. Methodically working with a metal nail file and doing her best to avoid damaging the intricately carved brass key plate that surrounded the lock, she managed to unbolt the trunk after a week of trying. To her delight, the trunk did contain a treasure of sorts: arranged neatly inside were embroidered handkerchiefs, beaded handbags, lacy blouses, dainty lingerie, fashion accessories like gloves and scarves, and little squares of silk. There were thimbles and spectacles, old letters, and postcards dating back to the 1920s, even homemade Valentines.

Sandra marveled at the find. Though its value in terms of

dollars and cents was negligible, as a writer she recognized the intrinsic worth of these mementos. Somebody's history was locked inside the trunk, somebody's story, long forgotten, never told. She has kept the trunk throughout the years, leaving its contents intact out of deference to both its original owner as well as to the symbolism it suggests. That decision mirrors Sandra's life as well because she also has a story locked deep inside her soul.

For decades the story lay dormant, like faded relics in an antique trunk. Only recently, though, has Sandra found the "key" that has helped unlock her story, and that key seems to be related to a decision she made a few years ago to write her memoir. Though the award-winning author has been successfully writing fiction for almost thirty years, she seems compelled, almost duty-bound, to explore her own history.

Even in the middle of a conversation, she'll abruptly get up from the table, excusing herself for a moment so she can retrieve her notebook from the other room. "I have to write that thought down," she calls out as she disappears down the hall, "before I forget what we were just talking about."

Before she forgets. There's always something new to discover, some hitherto unexplored aspect of her story that may be worth telling, if not now, then some day, and if not in writing, then perhaps in the conversations she has with people every day.

You see, there was a time—once upon a time—when Sandra Benitez told no one her secrets. Now she is done with secrets, especially the one she carefully guarded for most of her life.

The Early Years

Sandra spent her first fourteen years moving from place to place in Latin America with her Midwestern father from Missouri, her Puerto Rican-born mother, and her younger sister, Anita. Because her father was a Military and Agricultural Attaché at the American Embassy, the family relocated often, living in Mexico City and El Salvador, where they settled in an agricultural experimental station that had been ceded to the United States government and was now unoccupied. The expansive property had been neglected, but it didn't take long to restore the estate to its original splendor.

In her memoir, Sandra describes the property as lush and exotic—a veritable Eden. It was a time of relative peace in El Salvador, but in the tummy of a little girl named Sandilla (Sandy), it was a time of turmoil.

"I started getting sick when I was about five years old," the sixty-seven-year-old author said recently, "but I wasn't diagnosed with ulcerative colitis until I was thirty. I suffered mostly from constipation. There was a lot of bleeding and mucous. I did have bouts of diarrhea, sometimes four or five times a day, but it was terribly painful because of the inflammation in my rectum, which is where my disease was located." She would spend long hours every day sitting and straining on the toilet, yet in spite of her efforts, Sandra would frequently go days without a bowel movement.

Nevertheless, she seldom discussed her bathroom travails, not even with her family, and particularly not with her mother, who also suffered from various stomach ailments. Once when Sandra was eight, she discovered a bump in her rectal area, which she later learned was a hemorrhoid. Rather than telling her mother, she informed one of the household servants. In retrospect, she finds this self-imposed reticence incomprehensible. "It's amazing how people don't like to talk about this subject," she said. "I mean, think about it. Everyone has to poop! If we don't, we'll die! But to talk about it is a no-no."

These days, Sandra Benitez has no problems using words that most people find offensive. She has somehow been freed from the social restraints that for so long kept her muzzled. "When you're sick with something like a migraine headache, or maybe a shoulder pain, these are things you can talk about," she said. "But when you're sick with something that has to do with sitting on the toilet, nobody wants to discuss this. People don't like talking about bodily functions and are repulsed by anything that has to do with feces or the anus or the rectum. They'll talk about anything else, but those words are taboo. I'm talking here about shame. I felt shame because I had to use the bathroom frequently. And I was stuck in that shame for most of my life."

Though her family was aware that something was wrong with Sandra, they attributed her stomach problems to the fact that she was the "sensitive" one in the family. She admits to being an anxious child, resulting in a propensity toward perfectionism and overachievement—character traits that she speculates began in early childhood and persist to this day.

Over time she has learned enough about her disease to understand that personality traits do not in themselves cause ulcerative colitis. She does concede, however, that anxiety may have exacerbated her problems. "I believe I was more ill because I held things inside, literally, in the sense of being constipated, and emotionally in the sense that I never talked about my illness. Much later I would come to realize that neither of these habits was healthy."

When she was fourteen, Sandra moved from El Salvador to America to live with her paternal grandparents on their dairy farm in Missouri. The contrast between her pampered life in El Salvador, complete with household servants and lavish parties, and her new life on a rustic farm, was startling. Though charming and pastoral, her grandparents' farm—even in the mid-1950s—didn't have modern conveniences like running water or indoor plumbing. Her first year there, the only toilet facilities were an outhouse or a porcelain pot, which she refers to as a "thunder bucket." The chamber pot was stored in bedrooms and used either at night or when the weather was bad.

Imagine being chronically constipated and having to choose between an outhouse and a bucket. Most people would balk. Not Sandra. She didn't protest, but she did adapt. She learned to "hold" it in, waiting until she could use the restroom at school or at a friend's house. "You have to understand how I perceived things," she said. "I was only fourteen. I was practically on my own. I was struggling to make sense of what was happening to my body. It didn't occur to me that I was seriously ill. It was just something that I coped with."

Compounding the situation was Sandra's sense that she had been "sent away." It was not uncommon for children of foreign diplomats to return to the States, go to school, and become "Americanized," but in the mind of a sensitive young teenager, such a move could be perceived more as banishment and less like opportunity. It is noteworthy that Sandra's younger sister, Anita, was also sent to live on the farm. Unlike Sandra, however, Anita did not view the experience as a type of exile.

"I think Sandra perceived it that way at first," explained Anita de Alvarez, who now lives in Florida with her husband. "But the truth is my father wanted us to see the way other people live. We were not wealthy, but we did have a good life. He felt it would be an eye-opening experience for us both. Sandra is very respectful and compliant, and she always wanted to please our parents. I am different. I'm very outspoken. I hated living on the farm. I told my father, 'I can't stand this! This is killing me! Do you want your daughter dead or alive?' When my father saw how really unhappy I was, he said, 'OK, Anita you can come home.' So I went back to El Salvador, but Sandra stayed and stuck it out in America. She put up a good front but kept things inside all those years. Maybe that's why she writes so well—to express everything she kept bottled up inside."

Part of Sandra's unwillingness to discuss her problems may also have something to do with her upbringing. "Growing up in the home of an American diplomat, we often rubbed elbows with the elite of the country," she said. "The women were always well-dressed, especially after five o'clock, when they'd put on nylons and heels. It was all about appearances. They wanted to look their best at all times. They were also very concerned about odor. My mother had almost a fetish about cleanliness and odor, so I think I picked up on this attitude very early in life. If we were at somebody's house and had to use the toilet, we would just hold it until we could go in the privacy of our own home. You can imagine how this played out on a day-to-day basis: women simply didn't talk about their bathroom routines in general and their elimination in particular."

Throughout Sandra's college years, her first marriage, the birth of her two sons, and her early career as a translator and International Liaison at Wilson Learning in Minnesota, she kept her secret well. Co-workers and friends had no idea what she was contending with every day—how she would rise two hours before leaving for work to give her enough time to sit on the toilet; how she furnished her bathroom like an office, complete with bookcase and telephone, so that she could conduct business while seated on the throne; how she would often have to fend off the powerful urge to defecate at unexpected and inconvenient times; how she would flee in panic to the nearest toilet; how she would double up in agony at times as what felt like razor blades passed through her body; and how she would lean her head against the wall in the bathroom and sob in humiliation.

They knew none of this. All they saw was the poised, confident, successful exterior that she presented to the world. One long-time friend who worked for Sandra as her administrative assistant at Wilson Learning said she wasn't even aware that Sandra had undergone ostomy surgery until after the fact. "She never complained," said Mary Setter Bock, who has known Sandra for thirty years and remains friends with her to this day. "She was always full of energy and was an enthusiastic and diligent boss. Learning about her story later made me feel guilty in a way. As a friend, maybe I should have known. But she was obviously determined to lead her life and overcome her obstacles on her own. It's a brave story, but a sad one, too. I feel bad that I didn't know and could never help her."

Sandra's second husband Jim Kondrick, agrees. The seventy-six-year-old marketing specialist and former journalist believes being the partner of someone who suffers from ulcerative colitis is a challenge all its own. "The kind of disease that Sandy has can be a solitary disease," said Jim, who originally hired Sandra at Wilson Learning and who now helps market her memoir. "At first you're not even aware that there's a problem. You know she's spending quite a bit of time in the bathroom, and you notice there's a lot of pain, but you're on the sidelines. For me, all I could do was stand by and watch Sandy go through these various stages. I did what I could to help, but she made it pretty much a solitary battle. Later, when she began to think about having the surgery, again, she made it a private decision. We discussed it a lot, what it would mean, the irreversibility of it, which was very scary. But in the end, it had to be her decision."

No Longer Holding Off

In 1994, at age fifty-three, Sandra Benitez finally decided to have the radical surgery that her physicians and her brother-in-law had been recommending for years. The surgery was a proctocolectomy and permanent ileostomy, which involved the total removal of both her rectum and her anus and the creation of an ileostomy to collect her waste. It was a huge decision, one that she admitted she resisted for far too long.

"I held off for years," she acknowledged, adding that the difficult choice is the same for many people who are confronted with the option of ostomy surgery. "You will do everything you can to hold on to your body parts," she explained, "even body parts that aren't working well and even those as ignominious as your rectum and anus. In the back of your mind you're always hoping the disease will go away on its own, or that a new medication will appear on the horizon which will solve all your problems."

Though she understands the complexity of the decision, she learned quickly that having an ostomy was *not* the end of the world but a new beginning, and that being an ostomate does not define her as a person. This revelation is what ultimately compelled her to tell her story. True, the period of recovery immediately following surgery was painful, and the emotional letdown afterward was very challenging. When she came home from the hospital, she found herself crying uncontrollably for long periods until Anita arrived from Florida to care for her. She admits it took some time before she could even look at her new stoma, let alone develop a routine for emptying and changing her bag.

In the beginning, the bag attached to her side eclipsed everything else about who she was. She even referred to herself as a BAG LADY, using capital letters to signify the importance of the bag's role in her life. But after she finished writing her memoir and was contemplating a title for the book, she settled finally on *bag lady*, deliberately using small caps to symbolically relegate the ostomy's significance to a place of lesser prominence in the list of who she is and what defines her. "We are not victims," as she writes near the end of her memoir. "Bag-wearing is not our identity."

It has taken Sandra Benitez nearly a lifetime to be free from the shame of her illness, to reveal her secrets, to open the trunk of her life, as it were, and tell her story. When she decided to apply to the Great Comebacks program several years ago, it was not because she felt she was deserving of any kind of recognition or award, but simply because she had finally accepted herself for who she really was.

"A comeback has to do with coming back to who you are, not what others think you are," she said. "That's why the phrase 'great comeback' is so wonderful. It's coming back not just from surgery but from all the blows life dishes out. If we're people who happen to have ulcerative colitis, or Crohn's disease, or colon cancer, that's part of who we are, but it's *not* everything. And if we happen to have an ostomy"—she paused for a minute and looked down at her side, where concealed beneath her dress was the stoma she now refers to as her little spout—"we have to embrace it and realize that the surgery has given us a second chance to live, to chase down our dreams, and to become all that we were made to become.

"Life is so special, and all of us who go through this surgery come to understand that. We are the lucky ones, and we want the world to know that we are changed, not because of the way we eliminate, but because of how much we now appreciate life, our loved ones, the simple pleasures that we used to take for granted . . . something none of us will ever do again."

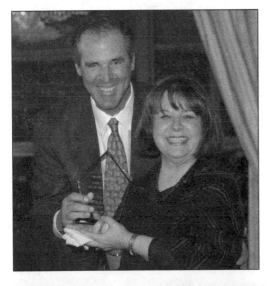

Gifted author Sandra Benitez was the recipient of the 2006 Central Region Great Comebacks Award.

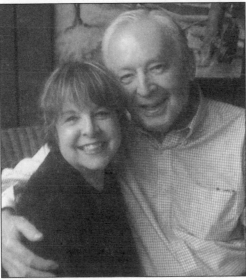

Sandra is continually touched by the response she receives from patients who read her book, and is supported in all she does by her husband, Jim.

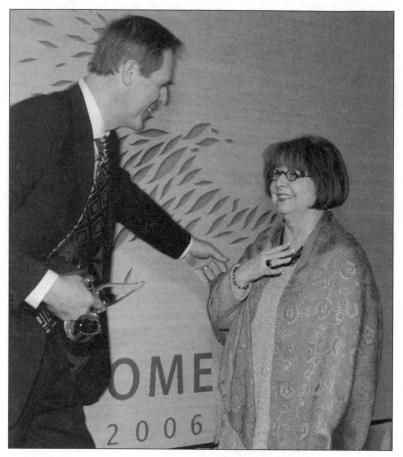

Sandra Benitez was momentarily at a loss for words as Rolf Benirschke announced her as the 2006 National Great Comebacks Award winner.

GETTING UP OFF THE MAT

"Once you've wrestled, everything else in life is easy."
—Wrestling legend Dan Gable

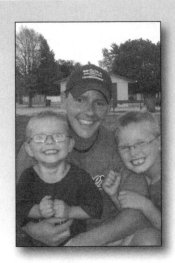

Rick Ellison

AGE: 34

HOMETOWN: Fond du Lac, Wisconsin

MEDICAL SITUATION:
A young wrestler discovers that no matter how hard he works inside the gym, he is no match for ulcerative colitis—until he undergoes ileostomy surgery and becomes a true champion.

People who don't understand wrestling fail to appreciate the appeal of a sport that involves manhandling one's opponent to the floor. Yet when you speak to wrestlers you discover a profound respect—bordering on reverence—for the sport. What is the allure of a pastime that some consider the highest form of unarmed physical combat and "the cruelest mistress in the world"?

It could have something to do with ancestry. Wrestling can be traced to ancient civilizations dating back thousands of years. Throughout history, everybody who was anybody wrestled. Greek gods wrestled. Henry the VIII wrestled. Plato wrestled. At least seven U.S. presidents wrestled, among them George Washington and Abraham Lincoln. There's even an account in the Bible of an angel wrestling with one of the patriarchs.

More likely, though, the sport has something to do with self-reliance. Wrestling is distinct from most other sports in that the athlete competes completely alone. He may be part of a team, but when he steps onto the mat, he depends on no one but himself. He will win—or lose—on his own efforts and imagination. If he's the last man standing with his arm raised in victory, it's because he alone made it happen.

It's this latter aspect of wrestling that attracted Rick Ellison to the sport when he was a little boy growing up in Fond du Lac, Wisconsin. Rick was eleven when he started wrestling seriously. "I was always the shortest kid in class," Rick explained, "and that is why I took to the sport. I also had a Southern accent and was living in Wisconsin, and that's when I found out that kids can be pretty ruthless. I learned early on that being athletic had advantages; if you're the quickest kid on the playground, you don't get teased. So at an early age, I got involved in all kinds of sports, and as I got a little older, wrestling became my favorite. In wrestling, being short doesn't matter because you're paired up against someone your own size."

As it turns out, "I found out I was pretty good at it," Rick said.

According to Rick's high school wrestling coach, it's hard to appreciate how good Rick really was because triumphant wrestlers a year ahead of him eclipsed his accomplishments. "In Rick's junior year, our team won the Wisconsin State Wrestling Championship," said Larry Marchionda, whose high school teams always ranked in the top five in the state. "Rick was on the junior varsity squad that year, and he went an astounding 72-0, but all the attention went to the varsity boys who won State. Ironically, it was Rick's work ethic that actually contributed to these boys' success. You see, every day he would stay in the practice room and push those older boys to excel. He was relentless and just wouldn't quit."

Rick concedes that hard work and discipline have always been important to him. "I'm a very goal-oriented, driven guy, almost to the point where it's not safe," he admitted. After wrestling practices, which even his high school coach acknowledges were grueling, Rick would continue training, going out late at night and on weekends to run. He especially enjoyed jogging in bad weather—

one time he even went out during a blizzard—because he knew there was little chance his opponent would be out training at that time. "My mindset was *this is my chance to gain ground, to get an edge over my opponent.* I believed that whatever I could do to get an extra step on everyone else was critical. It was my way of survival."

Rick's wrestling team qualified for State his senior year. His personal goal was to win the state championship in his weight class, go out on a high note, and retire from wrestling. Somehow, though, he drew the defending champion in the first round and barely lost. Disappointed but not undaunted, he reassessed his goals and decided to wrestle in college. "If I couldn't win State in high school, I wanted to be All-American in college to make up for it," he explained. He was well on his way to achieving this goal when unanticipated circumstances interrupted his plans once again.

Grabbing Hold Fast

Rick's first year wrestling as a freshman at the University of Wisconsin-Oshkosh got off to a slow start when injuries prevented him from finishing out his first season. He took a medical redshirt that year and started up again in 1994, his sophomore year. He was gaining muscle, bench pressing twice his weight, winning matches easily. He had also begun dating Abby, a former high school wrestling cheerleader also attending UWO. Abby was nineteen. Rick was twenty. Things were going well—and then he got sick.

Rick remembers when his digestive troubles came seemingly out of nowhere. "When it took hold, it took hold pretty fast," he said, referring to sudden and frequent bouts with cramping, diarrhea and bleeding that would eventually be diagnosed as ulcerative colitis. At first he thought he was experiencing symptoms related to his diet. "Wrestlers don't follow the best of diets," he explained, pointing out that wrestlers often starve themselves to "make weight," and then gorge themselves after weigh-in with high fat, greasy foods.

Consequently, in the early stage of his illness, Rick kept his symptoms to himself. His relationship with Abby was too new—he wasn't sure he was ready to talk about something this personal with her. He didn't want to burden his parents, and he wasn't about to tell his coach or teammates and risk spoiling another promising season.

Hoping the symptoms would disappear on their own, Rick kept his mouth shut and continued to wrestle. But instead of his symptoms disappearing, his condition worsened, and eventually he broke down and confided in his parents and his girlfriend.

Abby remembers the day Rick told her what was going on. They were heading back to the campus after visiting their hometown. "He knew he needed to see a doctor, but he didn't have any health insurance," she said, adding that Rick's parents had financial struggles of their own at the time, which is another reason why Rick didn't want to burden them.

Abby convinced Rick to see a doctor anyway. "They prescribed drugs to treat Irritable Bowel Syndrome, which helped for awhile, but then he'd get sick again. So he'd go back and they'd prescribe different drugs. Each time he would get better and think it was the last time, but he'd get sick again."

This went on for two years. Rick barely managed to scrape together enough money to pay for his prescriptions while continuing to work out. When his knees started to bother him—a side effect of the drugs—he worked out even harder. Yet it was becoming apparent to all his friends that his physical condition was deteriorating rapidly.

"Rick was obviously in a lot of pain," recalled Gary Flynn, one of his college roommates. "He was taking prednisone, so his face was bloated and splotchy, and his knees bothered him a lot. One day he walked into the room and literally collapsed onto the floor. I think the prednisone had worn away the cartilage in his knees, and he was pretty much walking bone on bone." Gary and his roommates picked up Rick, carried him to the car, and drove him to the hospital.

Abby recalls a similar crisis. "We had been dating about a year, and we still didn't know what was wrong," she said, knowing from their very first date that she would eventually marry Rick. "One day he came over to my apartment so I could take care of him. I remember it was almost midnight, and he was spiking a fever. My roommate wasn't there, and I wasn't sure what to do. I had put in a call to the ER and was waiting for a doctor to call back. I went to check on Rick, and I found him passed out on the floor."

During this period, when Rick was dealing with both the physical aspects of his illness and his anxiety over finances, something else was troubling him even more. His entire life had been characterized by seemingly endless reserves of strength, where he could run as far and lift as much as he wanted. Sports had defined him when he was growing up. Even his mother laughs as she reminisces about Rick's teenage years. "It was non-stop," Diana Ellison said, referring to the fact that all three of her sons were involved in all kinds of sports. "They'd hang up one set of shoes and take up the next."

Now, though, he was having a hard time keeping up with the guys on his college wrestling team. Fear of losing his identity as an athlete drove him to push himself even harder. The mindset that caused him to excel in high school kicked in—*I can beat this guy.* He resolved to do what he had always done when he needed to gain an edge over his opponent: push himself even harder. And so, when everyone else had gone home after practice to shower or relax, Rick would slip back outside and run stadium steps or sprints around the local park. Hard work had never failed him before—why should it fail him now?

One day, near the end of a regular practice, he was running steps in the stadium with his teammates. On this particular day he struggled more than usual. "I felt like I was ninety years old," he said, remembering what would become a defining moment in his life. "So I closed my eyes and visualized myself sprinting with all my might. I could see myself passing everyone else. But when I opened my eyes, instead of leading the pack, I was among the last. Just then, someone passed me. And it wasn't just anyone—it was the heaviest guy on the team. I'm the 118-pounder, the smallest guy on my team, yet our heavyweight was passing me."

It was too much. He threw his headgear against a wall, shouted, "I quit!" and broke down sobbing. "It wasn't because I couldn't keep up with everyone else," he said, trying to explain the significance of that moment. "It was a complete and total upheaval of my identity. Hard work had always been my way of surviving. Now I no longer had control. There was *nothing* I could do to make this thing go away."

The final indignity came during a wrestling match not long after this episode. Rick had informed his coach that this would probably be his final match—a match that Gary Flynn remembers vividly. "Under normal circumstances, Rick could have torn his opponent apart," Gary said. "Even in his weakened condition, he was ahead by six points! But then his opponent tight-waisted him, which is when you reach around your opponent's stomach and hold him in a vise-like grip. You could tell Rick was in excruciating pain, and from that point, his opponent just picked him apart. It was very difficult to watch."

Evidently, Rick's coach thought so, too, because he called off the match. Throwing in the towel was not the way Rick wanted his wrestling career to end, but there was nothing he could do to change that. The match was over, and his opponent was awarded the win. It would be the last time he wrestled at the collegiate level.

Eager to Get Off the Mat

Overwhelmed by what was happening, Rick decided to visit his parents, who had moved to Alabama, during spring break. On the last night of his visit, he became violently ill. His mother, Diana, relays the story: "Rick was eager to get back to school, but he began hemorrhaging and hallucinating. He was in so much pain, but he wouldn't let us take him to the hospital. Finally, when his fever reached 105, I couldn't stand it anymore, so we rushed him to the emergency room. They had to admit him because he was bleeding so badly."

It was during this hospital stay that Rick met the physician who would literally save his life, Dr. Steven Weinstein. The surgeon had heard through the grapevine about Rick. "He would come in every evening and talk with Ricky," his mother continued. "Eventually he convinced Rick that if he didn't have surgery, he would literally bleed to death."

The surgery Dr. Weinstein recommended was called an ileal pouch reconstruction, a fairly new procedure at the time that would involve two separate hospitalizations. The first procedure would remove Rick's colon and create a temporary ileostomy, and second would create an internal pouch, called a J-pouch, that would be reconnected to the rectum and eliminate the need for an external stoma.

The surgeon explained in detail what would be involved and patiently answered all of Rick's questions. "He made it seem so normal," Rick recalled. "He was very frank and honest about what it would be like to have an ostomy, and he explained that I would be able to do literally anything I wanted to after the operation. At first I found that hard to believe until I learned that he had had ostomy surgery himself. He made it seem as if wasn't a big deal."

Later, Rick's Uncle Richard, who was like a second farther to Rick, shooed everyone out of Rick's hospital room, sat down on the bed, and told him in no uncertain terms to have the surgery.

Rick knew his uncle was right, but he had no health insurance. His medical bills had grown so large that he wasn't sure he could ever pay off the debt. He decided he needed to talk things over with Abby before committing to the surgery. He even went so far as to purchase a plane ticket back to Wisconsin after he was released from the hospital.

But the night before his flight, Rick suffered another relapse and began hemorrhaging badly. He briefly considered not telling his parents and flying back to Wisconsin anyway, but common sense got the better of him. He crept into his parents' room, woke them up, and told them he couldn't do this anymore. Rick knew he needed to have the surgery.

Sometimes, a state will pay for the medical expenses of residents who don't have the resources to pay for life-saving procedures. Unfortunately, Rick was hospitalized in Alabama—not his home state—so there would be no money from the government. This, however, did not prevent Dr. Weinstein from proceeding with the surgery.

Remarkably, the surgeon waived all his fees, as did the anesthesiologist, but the hospital did not waive its fees. While he was recovering from his first surgery, a representative from the hospital's finance office repeatedly entered his hospital room, asking how he planned on paying for his hospitalization. Rick was too ill to discuss finances. His mother ended up threatening to call a lawyer if the financial representative didn't stop harassing Rick.

Several months later, when Rick tried to schedule his follow-up surgery, the hospital refused to admit him because of his outstanding debts. He didn't know what to do. He needed the second operation. He picked up the phone and called Dr. Weinstein.

When the surgeon heard what had happened, he was livid. Ten minutes later, the hospital called Rick back and admitted him. Once again, Dr. Weinstein waived his fees. "I don't know if he ever recovered his expenses," said Rick shaking his head with appreciation. "He knew I'd never be able to pay him back. I owe that man my life."

At the time of his surgery, Rick's weight had dropped to 109 pounds. The muscle loss in his legs was so severe that they looked like someone's arms, as Abby put it. After his surgery, Rick couldn't cross the room unassisted. He used a cane to hobble around his parents' living room and a wheelchair if he went anywhere else. When he felt a little stronger, he managed to venture down the driveway to the sidewalk and back, but even that was a challenge. "One time, my mom actually caught me before I fell because I couldn't lift my leg over a crack in the sidewalk," he explained.

The idea of competing in sports again wasn't even in Rick's thinking—his sole objective was simply to try to walk again unassisted. But then he stumbled on a magazine story that talked about others who had survived similar surgeries and gone on to play professional sports. The article talked about Rolf Benirschke and Chris Gedney, both of whom returned to play football in the NFL.

At the time, the idea of ever getting that healthy again seemed amazingly far-fetched, but it was all the encouragement this fierce competitor needed. Rick set small goals and achieved them: first, he'd walk to the mailbox next door, then to the end of the block, then down the street to the library. Each day he walked a little farther, each day a little faster. Soon he began jogging.

Coming All the Way Back

One year after his surgery, Rick returned to school and began working out again in earnest. That same year, two significant things happened; he and Abby became engaged, and his former high school wrestling coach hired him to be his assistant coach. This was not a trivial or token offer, Rick points out, because assistant coaches actually work out with the team on a regular basis. "I was wrestling some of the best high school wrestlers in the state," he explained. "That was when I realized I was back."

Five years after his surgery, Rick completed his first marathon. Since then, he has run eight marathons, won the Lake Geneva Half Ironman relay, and completed his first solo Half Ironman triathlon and his first Ultra Marathon. He also just finished his second Half Ironman, cutting twenty-five minutes off his previous time.

Importantly, he has not forgotten the debt he owes to the man who didn't charge him a dime for saving his life. Rick was never able to repay Dr. Weinstein in dollars and cents, but to this day he continues to "pay it forward" by volunteering with the Crohn's and Colitis Foundation of America and doing everything he can to be a role model and encouragement to others who face similar life-threatening surgery. Currently, he is the Wisconsin Run Coach for the Crohn's and Colitis Team Challenge Half Marathon Team, which sponsors a Half Marathon every year to raise both awareness and funds for the CCFA.

Though Rick did stop wrestling competitively, two years after his surgery he decided to enter "The Old Timers Tournament," an adult wrestling event in Fond du Lac. The evening after the tournament, Rick retreated to a quiet room in his house and penned a special thank you letter to his surgeon, the man who wouldn't give up on him and who had saved his life—for *free.*

Tucked inside that letter of appreciation was the first place medal Rick had just won that day, a token payment to be sure, but a symbol of the rich life that he had regained.

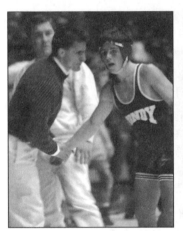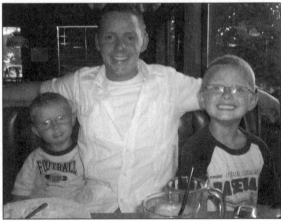

Rick Ellison, a star wrestler in high school, tried to compete in college until digestive woes forced him to throw in the towel. After all Rick has gone through, you can be sure that he will pass along his love of wrestling and his passion for life to his sons.

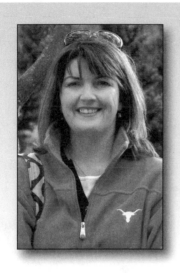

Julie Vaughan

AGE: 37

HOMETOWN: Plano, Texas

MEDICAL SITUATION:
Stress and an unhappy marriage have
family members believing that her
Crohn's disease is all in her head . . .
until the truth comes out after
submitting to ostomy surgery.

J ulie Vaughan describes herself as a "glass half empty" type
of person. By that she doesn't necessarily mean she's
pessimistic. If anything, she's what some might describe as
melancholic.

"By nature, I tend to see the worst-case scenario in most
situations," she explained. "I'm especially hard on myself. I worry a
lot, and I have a propensity toward depression. At one point, I
actually did suffer from clinical depression. So yes, for me, the
'glass' does tend to look half empty most of the time."

It was Julie's melancholic predisposition that muddied the
waters when she began exhibiting symptoms of Crohn's disease in
her early twenties. "I was about twenty-three when I began to get
sick, and at first I assumed it was all in my head," said the former
teacher and school librarian, now thirty-seven-years old. "I was
under a lot of stress, personally and professionally. I had just
finished college at the University of Texas and had decided to move
to Arkansas to be near my then-boyfriend. Since I was one credit

short of getting my teaching credential, I couldn't get a teaching job, so the first year I ended up subbing and waiting tables. That was in May 1993. In December I got married and knew immediately it was a mistake. Even on the eve of my wedding I knew. But my perspective at the time was, *It's too late, I'm already in this, I'm stuck.* My mom would call periodically and say, 'Are you sure this is what you want to do?' Other than those phone calls, I was completely cut off from my support system. If I had been surrounded by my friends and family, I probably wouldn't have gotten married."

The following year Julie landed her first full-time job teaching fourth grade in Springdale, Arkansas. The school year had barely begun when she began experiencing severe abdominal pain and cramping. "I wasn't sure what was causing the stomach problems, so I started experimenting with different foods," she said. "Eventually I figured out that if I just ate saltine crackers and drank water, I wouldn't cramp up. When you're in your twenties, you do crazy things, and for a while I lived on crackers and water rather than go see a doctor," she explained.

Part of Julie's reluctance to seek medical attention had to do with a sense that her problems might be stress-related, a suspicion reinforced by her anxious parents. "This is not a dig against my parents," said Julie, who quickly added that both her mom and her dad were extremely supportive during her illness. "But initially everyone blamed my stomach problems on my fragile emotional state at the time."

Julie's mother, Kathie Allison, acknowledges that in the beginning, before any of the family understood the nature of Julie's disease, she did attribute her daughter's physical problems to stress, and to some extent, she still wonders whether that unhappy time might have played a role in triggering the onset of Julie's illness.

"Julie entered into something that she knew was not good from the start," said Kathie, referring to her daughter's first marriage. "It got to the point where food became her enemy, which made me automatically think of eating disorders." Later on, one of Julie's physicians would suspect the same thing, and he would even say as much while treating her. So practically from the word "go" Julie struggled not only with the physical symptoms of Crohn's disease but also with self-reproach and depression.

Julie finally sought medical attention from a gastroenterologist in Arkansas and underwent a colonoscopy in April 1995. Test results revealed Crohn's disease, an autoimmune disorder that causes the lining of the digestive tract to become swollen and inflamed. The doctor explained that Julie's immune system was essentially attacking her intestines, which accounted for the severe cramping and excessive diarrhea. Julie found the news both welcome and overwhelming.

"When he returned with the results of the colonoscopy, I have to admit I actually felt relieved," she recalled. "At least I had a name for my problems—it wasn't all in my head." At the same time, she knew nothing about Crohn's disease. Inquisitive by nature, she began researching the disease, reading everything she could find and seeking out people who could flesh out the subject on a personal level.

Meanwhile, Julie's doctor started her on steroids. To minimize the side effects, he prescribed pulse dose rates, which, in layman's terms, refers to taking high doses of a strong medication for short periods of time and then suspending the doses before the body becomes dependent. Yet even the regulated quantity made Julie's life miserable.

"Steroids cause you to retain water, and they can also stimulate your appetite," she said. "There would be some days when I'd literally have to urinate all day long. Other days I'd stop off at Fat Boys Barbeque and order an entire meal after school, get home and eat another complete dinner, then wake up in the middle of the night *still* dreaming about food. Not only that, steroids made me extremely irritable. The slightest sounds and sensations grated on me. I guess you could say I was just a hyped-up version of myself and felt like I had little control of myself when I was on the drugs."

In a Tailspin

In spite of the drug therapy, the cramping and diarrhea persisted, and Julie continued to lose weight, at one point actually dropping fifteen pounds in three weeks. Somehow she made it to the end of the school year, but rather than taking time off to rest, she decided to teach summer school. Getting by primarily on a diet of Rice Krispie marshmallow treats ("For some reason, those sat well with me," she explained), she finished the summer in a tailspin. The chronic cramping and diarrhea, combined with stress at home and work, had left her reserves completely depleted both physically and emotionally. Not ready to leave her husband but desperately needing a break, she packed her bags and headed back to Texas.

Once she arrived at her parents' home in Hereford, she went into a funk. "I wouldn't get up off the couch, and I didn't go anywhere," she explained. "I had no interest in showering. I couldn't keep food down, and my parents were beside themselves, as you can imagine."

Julie's aunt and uncle, who happened to be doctors, dropped by one day to check in on their niece. It was immediately apparent to them, that in addition to her stomach ailments, Julie was also exhibiting signs of clinical depression. They strongly encouraged her to seek help and make an appointment with the hospital where they worked in nearby Amarillo.

On their recommendation, Julie followed through. She didn't know it at the time, but she was about to butt heads with a doctor whose brusque demeanor would inadvertently goad her into summoning up the personal resolve to get the care she needed.

The doctor was a large, commanding fellow, remembers Julie's mom, and he took no guff. "I don't think he necessarily did anything wrong," Kathie said. "He put Julie on steroids, which is often the first step in treatment, but he didn't really discuss the options with

Julie, and that didn't sit well with her. Julie has a mind of her own, and she just didn't want to take them. He became very angry when she challenged him, and that was where the problems started."

Julie doesn't disagree with her mom's recollection, though she does provide a slightly different spin. "When I visited this doctor as an out-patient, he said he would start me on steroids and explicitly warned me of the dangers of stopping once I'd begun. I understood the risks and agreed, but by the time I got home, I'd already made up my mind *not* to take them"—a minor detail she neglected to mention to the doctor.

"I guess you could say my response to him was passive-aggressive. I had no intention of taking the drugs, but I didn't want to challenge his authority. When I returned for a follow-up visit and he discovered I wasn't taking them, he assumed I had ignored his warning and exploded. He just laid into me. I understand his anger—he thought I had endangered myself. But he didn't have to say the things he did in front of my mom and the nurses. He really *shamed* me."

Julie, who admits she's "not very good in the moment," endured the tongue-lashing in silence. Afterward, she admitted herself into the hospital for a two-week period of "bowel rest" and observation, but her now-volatile relationship with the doctor remained was a problem.

"He would begin his rounds at six in the morning, enter my room, switch on the light, and say things like, 'What's wrong with you? Why aren't you getting better? Are you anorexic or bulimic, or is there something you're not telling me?' " she recalled. "It was taking me all night to fall asleep, so to suddenly be wakened up in such a rude manner was very hard for me. I could barely formulate a complete sentence to respond, and at that point, I had so little self-esteem that I couldn't possibly be an advocate for myself."

It's apparent the memory of this doctor still grates her. Julie admits that in the years since, she's run into him on a few occasions, and each time she sees him, she experiences almost a visceral reaction. But slowly over time she's managed to put the experience into perspective. She believes it helped shape her into the more confident, assertive, and informed patient she has become. "I've learned to appreciate what it means to be a partner in one's own health care. I interview and choose my doctors differently now, realizing I don't have to take that kind of treatment. I have rights as a patient."

Julie credits one of her nurses during that early hospital stay for helping to drive this lesson home. "By the end of the second week of bowel rest, it was clear I wasn't getting any better. This doctor wanted to repeat the *whole* battery of tests I'd already been through, including a colonoscopy. To tell someone in my condition that you need to scope them again is just about the worst thing you can say. Besides the physical trauma of getting scoped, you also have to drink this saline solution to clean out your intestines in preparation, and my bottom was already raw from constant diarrhea. At the time, I felt like I had no choice but to do what the doctor said.

"So, I was up all night using the toilet, and each time I went I got more and more angry and upset. At one point in the middle of the night, this nurse came in with the last dose, but for me, it was the last straw. I started crying hysterically and said there was no way she could make me drink it. To my surprise the nurse remained calm. She set the glass on a table and said, 'You do not have to drink this.' Then she explained that the doctor would come to scope me in the morning and that if I was not cleaned out, I'd have to go through it all again, but the choice was mine. Then she left."

For Julie, the words were heaven-sent—an epiphany. "I felt like that doctor had me backed into a corner with no options, but when the nurse let *me* decide whether to drink the solution or not, that empowered me. The decision was *mine*—no one could make me drink that vile stuff and force me to go through another colonoscopy. I felt liberated. I picked up the glass and drank. Naturally, I vomited it right back up. But I drank it on *my* terms. That nurse became one of the unsung heroes in my life."

Julie had one more epiphany before she left the hospital in Amarillo. Her husband came out from Arkansas to visit her, and they spent the afternoon talking about their marriage. Midway through the conversation, she had a moment of clarity when she knew in her heart that the marriage was over. But it would still be another year before she would have the courage to act on her decision—and even longer before she would be guilt-free.

She returned to Arkansas and taught one more year, and she even attempted marriage counseling before finally calling it quits. In May 1996, Julie moved back to her parents' home for the summer and began divorce proceedings.

Seeing Emotional Improvement

After her divorce, Julie moved into an apartment in Amarillo and found a job teaching special education. She also enrolled in an online Library Certification program, which her parents offered to finance. Though still battling Crohn's disease, she began to improve emotionally.

She reconnected with old friends, including James Vaughan, whom she had met back in college. James lived in Plano, and the two picked up their friendship where they had left off. It wasn't long before they began a long-distance courtship that had them flying back and forth between Amarillo and Dallas.

Julie was adjusting to her new single life while James was just starting his career. Julie also began to search for a new doctor, and because of all that she had been through, she knew exactly what she was looking for and had extremely high standards. Above all else, she wanted to have a say in matters related to her health, including whether or not to take steroids.

In July 1998—during a record-breaking heat wave—James convinced Julie to move to Plano so they could close the distance between them and see more of each other. In October, he invited her to see a football game at the University of Texas, where they had met years earlier. She wasn't feeling well at the time, but he insisted.

Besides, he'd already attended one hundred consecutive Longhorn home games—how could they miss this one? Reluctantly, she agreed.

When they arrived at the campus, Julie and James got out of the car and headed toward the stadium, holding hands and admiring the beautiful architecture and the ancient oaks that dotted the rolling hills of their alma mater. Julie remembers noticing how James' hands shook and thought, "He must really be excited about this game—he's actually trembling!"

James escorted her to one of the main campus landmarks, a 307-foot tall tower, where they sat down. There, in the shadow of the tower, James suddenly dropped to his knees and proposed. Julie couldn't have been more excited, and they were married a few months later in January 1999. By the time they returned from their honeymoon, however, Julie's stomach problems returned with a vengeance.

Just about this time it began to dawn on Julie's family that none of this was her fault. James shed some light on the family's initial misapprehension. "At first, Julie's family felt that her tendency to worry was literally eating away at her," he explained. "They didn't so much blame Julie as believe that if she would *just quit worrying*, she'd get better."

Unfortunately, this is a fundamental misunderstanding many people, even some physicians, have about the nature of digestive diseases . . . just get rid of the stress in your life and get happy again, and you will start getting better. It has been categorically proven that this is *not* true. In Julie's case, despite her newfound happiness, her health didn't improve and actually deteriorated after she got married.

Two months after her honeymoon, Julie returned to her new gastroenterologist, Dr. Katherine Little, for another colonoscopy— this time accompanied her husband. After the exam, the doctor called James into her office and closed the door. The gastroenterologist seemed stunned and explained that both she and the colorectal surgeon, Dr. Robert Jacobson, had practically "fallen out of their chairs" during Julie's exam. Julie's colon was so constricted the doctor could not even pass a pediatric scope through the passageway. "I don't know how Julie's even been able to function all these months," she explained incredulously.

James was the one who broke the news to Julie when she woke up from sedation. Still groggy, she took one look at his normally affable face and thought, "I am in *so much* trouble." Not one to sugarcoat the truth, James was blunt. "It's not good. The doctor said your colon is so bad that he thinks you're going to need ostomy surgery. We can talk with Dr. Jacobson and ask for a second opinion, but it looks like that's the direction we're going."

Julie began to cry—a reaction James had expected. Of all the various options Julie had been exploring in how to manage her Crohn's disease, surgery was the one she had adamantly refused to even consider. She couldn't imagine living with a bag and ever being able to return to teaching or doing the things she loved. In addition, she was just married and this seemed just so unfair.

What James didn't expect—what *no one* expected—was how Julie would react to the news once the drugs wore off. After leaving the hospital a few days later, she began to fervently research ostomy surgery with such vigor that "she just *owned* it," he said. "I remember being so surprised because that is not how Julie normally handles things. But it was almost as if when she realized there was no other option, she made up her mind to deal with it. She became a different person."

Julie agrees that her response was out of character. "I think I was desperate enough at that point to finally get well that I was ready to try anything." After consulting with Dr. Little, he agreed that the surgery could be postponed until summer so she could finish out the school year.

This also allowed Julie to begin to prepare physically and mentally for what lay ahead. She dutifully drank her glass of Milk of Magnesia every night out of a crystal Ralph Lauren goblet tied in a pink ribbon—a present from her mother-in-law so she could drink it in style. She met regularly with her enterostomal therapy nurse, Linda Buchanan, to learn how an ostomy worked and even contacted a teacher from her school district who had an ostomy.

Unfortunately, that first experience with an ostomy nearly changed her mind. "She showed me her stoma and her pouch, modeled her bikini, and even talked about her sex life with her husband," Julie said. "I remember walking away from that first visit thinking, 'No, no, no, I do *not* want to do this!' " Julie even told James she was having second thoughts.

A few days later, they took a drive to the neighborhood where the teacher lived, ostensibly to look at houses on the market. When they pulled onto her street, the woman happened to be gardening in her front yard. "We passed her house, and there she was, in her Bermuda shorts and sandals, trimming rose bushes!" James said, 'Hey look, there she is! She had an ostomy, and she's working in the front yard!' "

They drove on without stopping, but the episode had a profound impact on Julie. "It was nothing dramatic or extraordinary—she wasn't climbing a mountain or running a marathon. She was just doing normal, commonplace things like clipping roses." Another epiphany? Perhaps. Whatever it was, that glimpse of an ordinary woman doing an everyday task won Julie over.

Comfort That She Needed

In June 1999, after a relaxing Memorial Day weekend spent in Texas with her family, the Vaughans drove back to Plano for the surgery, accompanied by Julie's mom. Oddly enough, of the three waiting for Julie to be wheeled off to surgery, James was the one worrying, not Julie.

There were tears, as well. Julie is particularly grateful for the empathy and sensitivity of her surgeon, Dr. Jacobsen. "He came in and noticed the emotion right away," she said. "He could have been all businesslike and undemonstrative, but, instead, he put his arm around my shoulder and said, 'It's hard, isn't it?' I said, 'Yes.' And he said, 'You know, it *is* hard.' That comforted me in a way I can't describe. He didn't trivialize the emotion. Instead, he acknowledged and affirmed it."

A final hug and off she went, leaving James and Kathie to fret. How would Julie handle life after ostomy surgery? Would she hate living with an ostomy bag? Would she worry about how she looked, or obsess over what people thought? Would she regress emotionally and struggle once again with depression?

They needn't have worried. Almost immediately Julie realized the surgery was a "good decision." Following a five-day recovery in the hospital, she went home and healed beautifully, and for the first time for as long as she could remember, she was free of the pain of Crohn's disease. What a blessing!

It helped that she was immediately surrounded by a cadre of friends, family, and professionals who couldn't wait to support her recovery and bolster her spirits. Her dietician, who also had a stoma, was constantly telling her ostomy jokes like this classic one: "Do you know what's the hardest thing about having an ostomy? It's finding shoes to match the bag!"

Visiting relatives begged to see her new stoma and rather than being repulsed, they were fascinated. "I was inundated with people who were supportive and positive," said a teary-eyed Julie. And with a husband who couldn't have been more compassionate, Julie's half-empty glass was now filling rapidly.

Then to add to her blessings, two years after surgery, Julie became pregnant with Annie—her "miracle child," as Julie's mom put it. "Having a child had always been Julie's dream," Kathie said. "The pregnancy was totally unexpected, and then to have such a wonderful, easy time of it even with her ostomy, was more than any of us could have imagined. And James has been remarkable. From the very beginning, he never turned away from any aspect of Julie's disease. He's been Julie's rock."

For his part, James still marvels at his wife's transformation.

"When she won the Great Comebacks award, she was a little surprised at first because she'd never done anything special or unusual like some of the other Great Comebacks winners," he explained. "But the great part of Julie's story is that someone who is not naturally positive has taken such an incredibly positive approach to what at first seemed like a very dismal situation.

"To me, that's what the Great Comebacks award is all about. It's about normal, everyday people just like Julie. There are probably a lot more people who won't be climbing mountains or running marathons after their surgeries but who *will* be gardening, raising children, teaching school, or working in libraries. Julie's is a story of a regular person with regular goals who does regular things. She is a person who battled her illness and her surgery and her personal demons of self-doubt and despair. Now she is back to being healthy *and* happy—someone who just happens to have an ostomy. I have seen her half-empty glass fill to overflowing . . . and I can't think of a greater comeback."

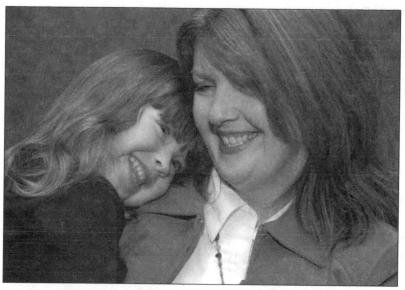

It took years for Julie Vaughan to realize that all her digestive-related troubles were *not* in her head and that ostomy surgery would return her to good health. Two years after her operation, she and her husband, Jim, were blessed with the birth of their "miracle child," Annie.

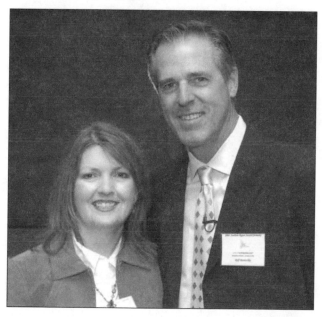

Julie was named the 2006 Southern Region Great Comebacks award recipient.

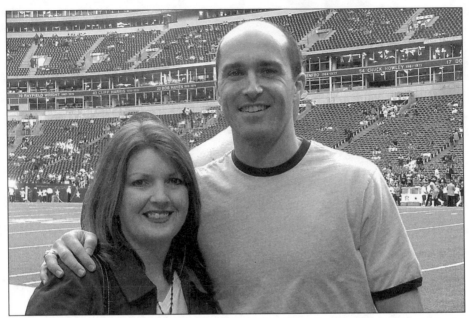

One of the benefits of being the Southern Region Great Comebacks Award recipient was the chance to spend time on the sidelines with her husband, Jim, before a Dallas Cowboys football game.

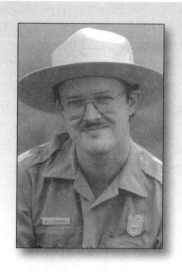

Bill O'Donnell

AGE: 49

HOMETOWN: Van Buren, Missouri

MEDICAL SITUATION:
While attending a school for
U.S. Park Rangers in his early twenties,
a young man stricken with Crohn's disease
is forced to have a permanent ileostomy . . .
and then prove he can still do his job.

H e begins his story where all good comeback stories begin: in the basement of a hospital kitchen, where we find him slopping mashed potatoes onto plates as they pass by on a conveyor belt, the only twenty-something guy among a couple of dozen employees, most of them women over fifty—a college dropout, a drifter, a self-professed bum.

"I'm a smart guy," Bill O'Donnell says today, reflecting on the sequence of events leading up to his illness. "But at the time, I didn't have a positive image of myself. I hadn't worked; I'd frittered away my father's college money; I'd quit school in my senior year at Ohio State. Here I was in a dead-end job, going nowhere. I admit it—I saw myself as a loser."

One day in particular stands out in his memory as a turning point. He was on lunch break, reading the newspaper in the cafeteria. One of his co-workers, a woman in her seventies named Mrs. Tucker, happened to be sitting nearby. His eye caught an ad for Ranger Training Academy. He started visualizing himself as a park ranger—the adventure, the outdoors, the wildlife, the bugs. He loved bugs. As a kid, he spent afternoons collecting insects in the woods, watching birds, damming creeks, building hide-outs. But there was this whole self-esteem thing. Could he rise to the challenge? Maybe. Then again, probably not. Park rangers are exceptional people. Muttering something to Mrs. Tucker about how he'd never be able to do anything that cool, he shoved the paper aside.

In a scene that might have been taken from a movie, Mrs. Tucker grabbed Bill's arm as he started to leave. There were no mincing words. "You go to that school," she said, jabbing her finger in his face, "and you make something of yourself." According to Bill, you ignored Mrs. Tucker at your own peril. Arguing with her was like arguing with your grandmother. All he could say was, "Yes, ma'am." He enrolled in the school within weeks of that encounter.

Hocking College sits on 2,300 acres of scenic countryside in southeast Ohio. The Ranger training program at the two-year college is designed to prepare students for a career in outdoor services, which can include everything from performing high cliff rescues and fighting fires to leading walking tours at nature centers.

A typical day at the campus might better resemble boot camp than school. "Rather than sitting in a classroom taking notes from a professor for a couple of hours," Bill explains, "you could spend an entire day on a specialized topic like Search and Rescue. Instructors are generally working professionals, like police officers or rangers on vacation, which adds a more real world sense than a lot of book material."

From the moment Bill set foot in his first class, he knew he had found his niche. Even so, there was no guarantee he would land a job once he finished his coursework. Most people vying for park ranger jobs not only have college degrees, but they also have several years of on-the-job training. Fortunately for Bill, one of his instructors happened to be the current Chief Ranger at Pictured Rocks National Lakeshore in Michigan's Upper Peninsula.

Because of Bill's limited experience, he could only be offered a volunteer summer job at Pictured Rocks. Even without a salary, it was the start he needed. And so it was that William "Bill" O'Donnell, barely twenty-five and fresh out of Ranger School, arrived in Grand Marais, Michigan, in June 1985, ready to embark on his career as a Park Ranger.

His residence for the summer was a bedroom on the second floor of an old Coast Guard Lifesaving Station, the first floor having been converted into a Visitor Center and Maritime Museum. He describes the building as a "tidy white two-story structure set right at the entrance to the harbor, with sand dunes spreading out between it and Lake Superior." Three others shared the bedroom and single bathroom, but Bill didn't mind. He pinned some posters on the wall beside his bed and walked over to the window, where he could see "the sweep of sand and water and sky that was austere and humbling." The self-described drifter was home.

He spent his first weeks doing various tasks in preparation for the museum's grand opening. Once the museum was open to the public, his work became somewhat more meaningful: staffing the information desk, issuing permits, helping with exhibit designs, doing research, assisting with sales. In his free time, he hiked the rugged shoreline and explored the forests of dark spruce and birch, craggy sandstone cliffs, and sculpted rocks towering nearby. "Lake Superior has a terrible sort of beauty," he says. "There's nothing as awesome as watching a storm roll in, whipping up the surf to rival any ocean."

Bill's not sure exactly when he first began to bleed "from places you're not supposed to bleed," as he put it in characteristic understatement. Since there were no other symptoms, he ignored the bleeding at first. Nothing was going to interfere with his dream of becoming a ranger. It wasn't long, however, before he began to experience some serious abdominal discomfort in addition to the bleeding. He finally confided in another staff member, a retired Air Force flight surgeon, who recommended that he try soaking in a bath daily. This posed a problem, as the communal bathroom contained only a shower stall and no tub. The ever-resourceful Bill, experiencing more and more pain, created a makeshift sitz bath using a large plastic basin, which doubled as a storage bin when not in use. Fearing discovery by his roommates (he did feel a little ridiculous, sitting in a plastic tub in the shower), he would soak at odd hours of the day—usually when people were out of the building—or late at night, while everyone else slept.

The soaking provided temporary relief from discomfort, but the bleeding didn't stop, and attempts to self-medicate were ineffective. The time had come to seek medical attention. Once again, though, his options were limited. Grand Marais had a population of about 350, with the nearest hospital about 100 miles away. There was a doctor who flew in to Grand Marais from a nearby town and set up a portable health clinic in the town hall every other week. Dreading what he knew would be an unpleasant and embarrassing exam, Bill reluctantly made his way to the community center.

A Doctor's Examination

To Bill, perhaps the toughest thing he's ever done was to pack his bags, bid farewell to his supervisor, climb into his '66 Dodge Coronet, and drive 600 miles in order to move back in with his parents in Stow, Ohio, wondering if he was going to be forced to give up his dream of becoming a park ranger.

The doctor who examined Bill in Grand Marais had diagnosed his problem as an abscess in the rectal wall called a fistula, which would require surgery. Back home in Ohio, Bill consulted his family physician, hoping to avoid surgery and treat his problems with medications. Within weeks, however, his family doctor referred him to a surgeon, who concurred with the original diagnosis and recommended surgery. Bill underwent the first of what would eventually be five surgeries—the last of which would result in a permanent ileostomy—embarking upon a painful medical odyssey that would take seven hospitalizations and several years spent bedridden in excruciating pain before his as-yet undiagnosed illness was under control.

He jokes about it now. "When they told me I had a fistula, I thought it was a river in Eastern Europe," he quipped. But even he concedes those early days were difficult, especially since he was not taking anything stronger than Tylenol to manage the pain.

"Looking back on those days," he said in an interview from his office at the Ozark National Scenic Riverways National Park in Van Buren, Missouri, where he works as an Education Ranger, "I can't imagine going through what I did without prescription pain medication. Now I'm a big believer in Demerol!" he adds, laughing. "But at the time, I would pop five or six Tylenol in my mouth and then soak in the bath for half an hour."

His days after that first surgery were spent reading, doing crossword puzzles, and watching television—mostly old reruns of "Leave It to Beaver" or "Eight Is Enough." (There was no cable or satellite TV in those days, let alone videos or DVDs at his parent's house.) Eventually he stopped reading altogether and just watched TV.

He stayed up late at night watching the original black-and-white episodes of "The Fugitive," which came on at 3:00 a.m. "I would lie in bed and watch TV until I was too tired to keep my eyes open," he says, realizing now that he was probably seriously depressed at the time. "All I could think was, *This is all there is, and this is all there ever will be. I'll never be a park ranger; I'll never get a job. I'm an invalid, a spectator. And I'm probably going to die.*"

Indeed, Bill's older sister Kathy says there was a point when their parents became so alarmed about their youngest son's condition that they actually purchased a cemetery plot for him. At the time, she explains, no one knew what was wrong with Bill. His condition worsened when the wound from the first surgery, which involved draining the rectal fistula, didn't heal.

So, six weeks later Bill was back in the hospital for a second surgery. He lost a significant amount of weight and was in constant pain. Then came the crisis: two months after his second surgery he got violently ill with an intestinal bug and was rushed to the hospital in metabolic shock. His father, also named Bill, remembers the day vividly. "I actually carried him into the emergency room, but nobody seemed to want to do anything," he said over the phone from his home in Ohio. "I admit I blew my top a bit."

Bill's memories of the crisis are murky: he does recall his father, "a blustery Irishman," complaining to an ER doctor about the doctors who weren't making an effort to treat his son. He remembers his dad running a red light en route to the hospital and the chaos of the ER, but not much else. "Honestly, quite a bit of that time is fuzzy to me," he said. "It wasn't drugs—they didn't give me any! Just pain and illness, I suppose, clouding the memory. Constant pain can really wear a person down. It's hard to describe." He slept for three days.

The near-death episode was a turning point. Until then, no one knew what was going on, and Bill still had not received a proper diagnosis. When it was over, a set of fortuitous circumstances ("My first doctor went on vacation") led Bill to a new doctor. This doctor diagnosed Crohn's disease, a chronic inflammatory illness of the intestines that, as Bill described it, literally eats away at the cells lining the intestines. Though the disease is incurable, a palpable sense of relief came over the O'Donnell family. At last they had a name for Bill's condition, and with a name, some options. The new doctor prescribed prednisone, which alleviated the symptoms for a time. Bill even found a job working at a state park near his home that summer.

Eventually, though, the symptoms returned, but this time, the O'Donnells were better informed. They drove to the Cleveland Clinic, about thirty miles from their home, and met "that Australian doctor"—as Bill Sr. put it—Dr. Victor Fazio. Little did they know that Dr. Fazio was a world-renowned colon and rectal surgeon and one of the kindest and most understanding doctors they could ever meet.

It was then that Bill learned about the possibility of ostomy surgery. On Dr. Fazio's strong recommendation, Bill received a temporary ileostomy in 1988 in order to give his diseased colon a chance to heal. But, as Bill tells it, "They connected me up again about a year later to see if I'd be continent, but unfortunately, I wasn't. I had hoped that I would no longer need an ostomy, but trusting in my surgeon's counsel, I finally accepted that I would wear this bag for the rest of my life."

In 1990 Bill went under anesthesia one last time and received a permanent ileostomy. Now, finally healthy and not willing to let any more life slip past him, he married his college sweetheart, Julie and, two years later, had a son. Bill is especially indebted to Julie, who in addition to putting up with a lot of his corny jokes ("He's got a great sense of humor," she concedes), has seen Bill through countless medical crises since his surgery.

"There was a time when I had the ambulance number memorized before 911 was established in our area, and when I could almost look at a calendar and predict that we'd have to call for an ambulance," said Julie, a former landscape horticulturist who now stays home to raise their son and volunteers part-time at a local thrift store. Julie, who has emergency first response training, can usually handle most crises on her own. Occasionally, though, Bill experiences what Julie calls a "blip on the radar screen" and what the doctors refer to as "Crohn's bug attack."

"Usually these episodes are related to an intestinal bug," Julie said, explaining that even something as relatively harmless as a stomach bug can cause Bill to quickly dehydrate and go into shock if it's not managed in time. "We're forty-five minutes to a small hospital and over an hour to a larger one, so sometimes we need to get him hooked up to an IV to prevent dehydration."

Fortunately, these crises are becoming less frequent and though traumatic, the family has learned to adjust. Even ten-year old Paul has grown used to the arrival of emergency vehicles. "Once, one of the ambulance drivers even said, 'If I'd known your son was awake, I'd have put the lights on for him,' " said Julie, who has gotten into the habit of baking brownies for the drivers after an ambulance run. "Basically you have to re-group for a week, and then get going again," she said smiling. "It's the nature of the beast."

Appreciative of Life

It's been nearly twenty-five years since those early days of slopping mashed potatoes onto plates in that hospital basement. Gone are the days spent lying on a couch, watching other people live their lives, and waiting for the show to end.

Since then, Bill's career as a Park Ranger has blossomed and provided enough adventures to fill an entire season of reruns. He's fought forest fires in Shenandoah National Park in Virginia; carried an injured young woman away from a burning car while working at Ozark National Scenic Riverways in Missouri; participated in a manatee rescue in the Everglades; and helped with rescue efforts in the aftermath of Hurricane Katrina. He's had run-ins with aggressive elk, growling bears and charging alligators. A trivia buff, he's appeared on *Jeopardy!* and *Who Wants to Be a Millionaire.* He's a wildlife photographer, an educator, an entrepreneur, an environmentalist, a writer . . . and a college graduate.

Bill tries to explain what the ileostomy has meant to him.

"After my surgery, I was giddy, almost nauseatingly cheerful," he says. "There was this exhilaration, like there was nothing I couldn't do. This experience—of going several years without walking, of the ordeal it was to just go from the bedroom to the bathroom, and then, almost miraculously, to have my health returned because of my ileostomy—has changed the way I live life. Being acutely aware of the possibility of dying, whether from Crohn's disease or by being hit by a truck, has made me realize the importance of experiencing every positive thing I can in life, letting nothing go undone and no day unlived. I've also realized I have a debt—a requirement to return this gift in some way by giving back to others who will walk the same paths I walked and who will wrestle with the same challenges I have."

He pauses, as if wanting people to understand, "I have a great life, and others can too if they just persevere."

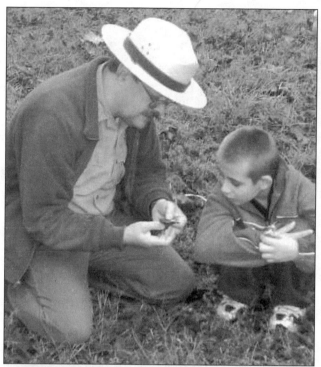

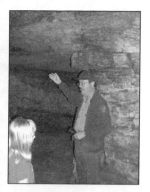

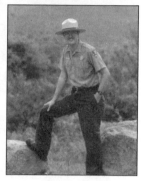

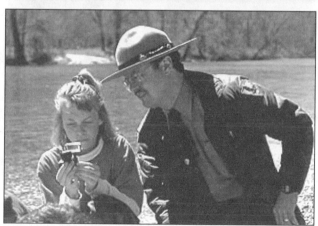

As a kid, Bill O'Donnell loved bugs and all things outdoors. He found that being a park ranger fulfilled all of his passions, and today he works at the Ozark Scenic Riverways National Park as an Education Ranger despite ostomy surgery that threatened his career.

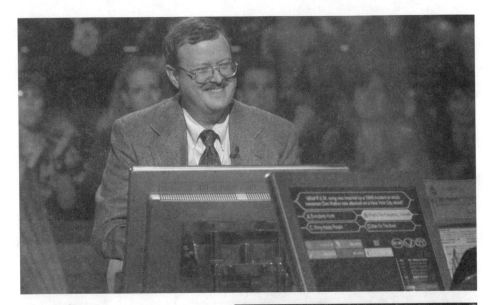

Always willing to try something new, Bill appeared on several game shows, including " Jeopardy!" and "Who Wants to Be a Millionaire."

Bill's favorite times are still spent with his son, Paul.

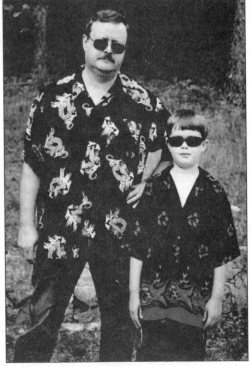

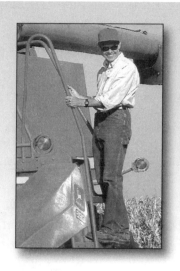

Charlie Grotevant

AGE: 66

HOMETOWN: Buckingham, Illinois

MEDICAL SITUATION:
A Midwest farmer battling
severe ulcerative colitis and
ready to give up . . . discovers a
whole new life after ostomy surgery.

O h, life on the farm . . . pastoral . . . even idyllic. Indeed, the word "farm" itself conjures up images of cozy houses with wraparound porches and white picket fences; charming barns filled with freshly reaped hay and grain; country roads lined with maple and birch, and dappled sunlight filtering through the branches while barnyard creatures strut and peck in the yard.

The earthy scent of fresh soil wafts on the warm summer breeze, stirred up by tractors churning sleepily in the distance. Horses, sheep, and cows graze in grassy pastures, and acres of sun-drenched wheat ripple gently beneath dazzling skies dotted with wispy clouds. Picture perfect, the farmer's life, right?

Not so fast. Though there may be some accuracy to this bucolic tableau, Charlie Grotevant will be the first to tell you that image and reality are often not the same.

"People who don't live or work on a farm seldom see the whole picture," said the sixty-six-year-old retired farmer from Buckingham,

Illinois, a small farming community in central Illinois. "Growing up on a livestock farm, a person was constantly walking in and around manure. The hot and sweaty jobs of baling and storing hay in barns and shelling corn from corncribs were always accompanied by lung-choking dirt. As with much of life, nostalgic moments captured in photos or people's memory are typically glamorized, while behind the scenes the jobs are often dirty."

Charlie, who grew up on a farm and has been farming for nearly his entire life, has seen the profession evolve from a time when farmers sold their milk and eggs locally to gigantic co-ops that are the hallmark of modern agribusiness today. "Farm life in the 1940s and '50s was a lot different from the way it is now," explained the lanky Kankakee County resident. "Back then, there was a lot of interaction with neighbors. When one farmer was baling hay, people from neighboring farms would often come and help get the hay into the barn. The next day, we'd all be at another neighbor's farm doing the same thing. Nowadays, agriculture is big business," he added, noting that at the peak of his career, he and his wife, Joyce, were farming 1,300 acres of corn, soybeans, and wheat. "With the advent of modern machinery and technology, you can farm several thousand acres today with no more effort than what it took us to farm a couple hundred acres when I was growing up."

That's not to say farming has gotten easier. Charlie is quick to point out that the physical demands of farming remain much the same as they have always been. "Even on a farm equipped with the newest and most efficient machinery, the behind-the-scenes activities are time-consuming and strenuous," he explained. "Activities like machinery maintenance, working in grain storage structures while transferring large quantities of grain, and handling livestock and livestock waste consume much of the time on today's farms."

And though Charlie concedes that farming is physically very demanding, he also believes the profession does have its perks. "You're outdoors every day, and you're close to nature, which is what I believe life is all about. Then there's the added benefit of being independent. On a rainy day, my wife and I could just get up and do what we wanted and not go to work. We didn't have to ask the boss," he says with a grin.

Charlie and Joyce Grotevant have been their own bosses for more than forty years, having embarked on their farming career in 1966, a few years after they got married. They spent their first three years of married life in Fort Devens, Massachusetts, where Charlie was stationed in the Army, before returning to Illinois and leasing a farm in Odell, the town where Joyce grew up. They farmed in that location four years before moving to a larger farm twenty miles east in Buckingham, where they currently reside.

In 1972, shortly after moving to Buckingham, Charlie began to experience symptoms of what would later be diagnosed as chronic ulcerative colitis. "In my childhood, I remember having stomach problems and irregular bowel movements, but it wasn't until I turned thirty that I first experienced serious pain and cramping," he said. "My general practitioner tried various medications, but none of them seemed to work. Eventually he prescribed prednisone, which is a steroid drug that has a soothing effect on the bowels but, unfortunately, has plenty of nasty side effects. The worst side effect for me was how it affected my personality. I don't think I was a very nice person to be around during those years."

Joyce agrees that those were difficult days for both of them. "Charlie's a very private person, and sometimes I wouldn't even know what was going on until it was really bad," she said. "And no, he wasn't pleasant to be around when it got bad. He would fly off the handle and holler at you and make things difficult and say everything was your fault."

Though Joyce took the brunt of Charlie's outbursts, she was mostly unfazed. "I knew he was hurting so I didn't give him any flak," she said, chuckling as she recalled how she deflected the worst of Charlie's outbursts. He was most irritable when his doctor prescribed cortisone enemas, and she was the only one around to help Charlie administer them. "He didn't like to have them done," she said with mild understatement.

"They hurt!" Charlie retorted. "You need to put the enemas right in the rectum to treat the sores. I tried to self-administer them, but I gave up on that. So I talked Joyce into doing them for me. Of course, I'd be in the throes of a flare-up at the time, so she'd be the only one I could holler at. But she'd get the job done, and I'd finally shut up and go to sleep. It's a shame, though, that my wife and kids had to absorb quite a bit of my mood swings and fits of anger," he admitted regretfully. "I blew up at them a lot."

At the time of the onset of the disease, Charlie and Joyce were farming over seven hundred acres of leased land, and Charlie was feeling quite a bit of stress—physically and emotionally. He did his best to cope in spite of the frequent episodes of cramping and bloody diarrhea, and he remembers many "bathroom" stops out in the field.

"It may be an exaggeration," he said, laughing, "but I figure during the years I was sick, I fertilized plenty of those crops with my own manure. I would instruct people working with me in the field not to come over if they saw the tractor stopped because I probably had my pants down. Just one more perk of farming," he joked. "I was much more fortunate than someone who works in a factory or office and has to hunt for a toilet. I could just drop my pants, do what I had to do, and then get back to work."

He laughs about it now, but Charlie acknowledges that he struggled quite a bit with depression back then. "There were days I thought I *would* die, and there were days I wished I would die," he said. He has since learned that mood swings and depression are common among people who suffer from inflammatory bowel diseases and especially those on medication.

"People I talk to pretty much tell the same story: in the depths of the flare-ups, they didn't want to live anymore and often even contemplated suicide. I admit to having similar thoughts. I wallowed in self-pity, sometimes for weeks at a time. I couldn't get myself focused on anything positive. I had this ruined body; I wasn't trained to do anything besides farming; and I was worried that that might all go away. I was concerned about our livelihood and credit my wife and three children for helping me get through all of that. Without them, I could not have gotten through my depression and might not be here today."

Things came to a head in September 1977, right around the time of the fall harvest. Charlie had lost a significant amount of weight, and his body was worn down by flare-ups that were increasing in frequency and severity. His doctor referred him to a gastro-enterologist, who diagnosed Charlie with severe ulcerative colitis and hospitalized him immediately. Charlie ended up staying in the hospital for two weeks, and it was during this stay that he began to learn more about his illness. One of the things he discovered was that while the disease could sometimes be managed with medications, the only real cure for ulcerative colitis was the surgical removal of the large intestine. He remembers telling a doctor at the time that he'd rather be dead than be forced to wear a bag.

Field Loss

September in the Midwest is when the corn harvest begins, followed shortly thereafter by soybeans. According to Charlie, timing is crucial during harvest season. Once the crops are matured, you need to gather them in as quickly as possible while the sun is shining to prevent field loss.

"Weather conditions, field conditions, and maturity of the crops determine what farmers do and where and when they do it on any given day during this season." Unfortunately, during the harvest season of 1977, Charlie Grotevant was not out in the fields reaping the harvest; he was lying in a hospital room sixty-five miles away, hooked up to an IV drip, fighting to stay alive.

In the meantime, word got out that Charlie was sick. "We didn't ask for help," Joyce remembers with a tear in her eye, "neighbors and family members just pitched in and helped with that year's harvest. One or two of our friends must've said something. Soon there were a dozen combines and all kinds of trucks and tractors out in our fields taking care of the crops. Even the fuel dealer showed up to fill up the vehicles. It was really quite a sight."

Joyce didn't tell Charlie about what was happening, but on the day she picked him up from the hospital to bring him home, all of the combines were still in the fields. "We arrived home late in the afternoon," he recalled. "I can still remember cresting the hill and seeing all those machines running in our fields doing all of this work for us. I couldn't believe it and just broke down in tears. I was so overwhelmed with gratitude."

Two years later on a Sunday afternoon in mid-November, Charlie was sitting in his living room watching football, one of his favorite pastimes. Since his hospitalization, he had been reading up on ulcerative colitis, familiarizing himself as much as he could with his disease and sorting through his options.

At this point, he still resisted the idea of surgery, but in Charlie's mind, it was evident that life with ulcerative colitis *and* life as a farmer were incompatible. Though he would experience periods of remission when he felt fine and didn't seem to need medications, inevitably there would be another flare-up and he'd have to get back on prednisone. This would send him again down a path of misery and despondency from the frustrating and embarrassing symptoms of colitis and the subsequent side effects of the drug. He knew this wasn't a life he wanted to live . . . but surgery?

As Charlie continued to research his disease, he ran across a story about a young placekicker from San Diego named Rolf Benirschke. He read about how Rolf's promising career in the NFL had been rudely interrupted by the very disease Charlie was struggling with, and how ostomy surgery had literally saved Rolf's life. The story made a big impression on Charlie, and on that particular November afternoon, it just so happened that Rolf's team, the San Diego Chargers, were on TV playing the Pittsburgh Steelers.

Charlie leaned forward and watched with interest. The Marine

Corps band had just finished playing the National Anthem, and the public address announcer was just introducing the captains for the game. One of the captains was Rolf Benirschke, the guy Charlie had been reading about and who had undergone ostomy surgery just weeks earlier.

Charlie watched as Rolf, dressed in white overalls and a team jersey draped over his emaciated frame, step haltingly onto the field and shuffle to midfield for the coin toss. Two huge linemen straddled him: defensive tackle Louie Kelcher and offensive tackle Russ Washington, veritable giants compared to the frail and ailing placekicker. While a capacity crowd of 52,000 fans rose to their feet and began to cheer inside Jack Murphy Stadium, halfway across the United States one man sat in silence in his living room chair, deeply moved by what he was watching.

Charlie kept track of Rolf's recovery over the next few years. He read how the San Diego kicker eventually regained his strength and resumed his football career in 1980 while wearing an ostomy pouch on his abdomen. He celebrated when he heard about Rolf's game-winning field goal in a dramatic playoff win against the Miami Dolphins in 1982, while still wearing that pouch.

At first, Charlie was impressed, but it wasn't long before he became inspired. Rolf's determination to overcome personal adversity and return to the game he loved had a profound impact on him. In May 1983, Charlie put on a pair of sneakers, donned some sweat pants, stepped out onto one of those charming country roads, and began to jog.

At first, he could barely run half a mile and hoped none of the neighbors were watching. Nevertheless, he persisted. He didn't run fast, but he did run farther and longer each successive day, and eventually he began to pick up speed. It wasn't long before his personal physician began to notice a change in Charlie's overall health.

"I was seeing the doctor about once a month, even when my colitis was in remission," Charlie said. "The nurse always took my blood pressure and heart rate during those visits, and each time I visited, the readings were a little better. It was obvious that the running was helping my body."

In September 1983, however, another flare-up put Charlie back in the hospital. This time Charlie's son, who was in college by then, came home to help Joyce and the neighbors with the fall harvest. It was then that Charlie finally realized that if he wanted to keep on farming, or continue any kind of active lifestyle, he would have to submit to ileostomy surgery.

"By the time I chose to have the surgery, I was ready. I was done with letting my life slip by in constant pain and uncertainty and was set to accept the challenge of wearing a pouch," he said, explaining the transformation from stubborn refusal to absolute certainty.

"Once I was convinced that the surgery would restore my health, the thought of wearing a pouch became a minor inconvenience. I read extensively about what it took to manage an ostomy and was prepared to handle the pouching systems. I finally realized that I needed the surgery, or I would have to do something different with my life. I chose the surgery and have never looked back."

Benefits Right Away

On November 10, 1983—the day he says his new life began— Charlie returned to the hospital one last time and had his large intestine removed. Four months later, just about the time the snow began to melt and patches of color started to appear along those picture-perfect country roads, he once again pulled out his sneakers and started jogging. He had seen the benefits of running prior to his surgery and decided that jogging would be a great way to get back into shape. After all, if Rolf Benirschke could come back and kick in the NFL better than ever, he reasoned, then he ought to be able to get back to running and farming.

His doctor cautioned him to ease into his training regimen slowly, but to Charlie, fresh air and sunshine became his drug of choice, as he put it. "Running was my way of celebrating a life free of illness, free of prescription drugs, free of pain. Sometimes I would recall the depression and discouragement I felt during those years battling colitis, and I remain determined more than ever to never to allow those feelings of self pity and uselessness to ever again dominate my life."

This is also the mindset that motivates Charlie to share his story with others who suffer from inflammatory disease like ulcerative colitis or who are facing ostomy surgery.

"I tell people it's not what happens to you in life, it's how you react to what happens," said Charlie, who now not only jogs for fitness but also races competitively. He proudly boasts that he's competed in more than nine hundred road and trail races and fifteen marathons—including the prestigious Boston Marathon— and has logged more than 41,000 running miles while wearing an ostomy appliance.

"One of the messages I try to share with people is that ostomies save lives and allow people to return to their passions. I encourage them to look at their ostomy as a tool that gives them a second chance at living, and to recognize that without it, they could be six feet under and never again see the beauty of an open road or feel the warmth of a sunny day."

Joyce, who stood by Charlie during the bleakest years, agrees. "Life's been wonderful since he had his surgery twenty-five years ago. Charlie has such a different perspective on life today . . . and he's a lot more fun to live with!" she says with a smile.

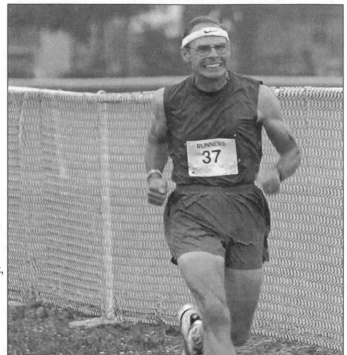

If you're running in the senior division, you don't want to be competing against Charlie Grotevant, who has run in more than nine hundred road races since his ostomy operation.

It was difficult for Charlie's wife, Joyce, during the early years of his battle with ulcerative colitis, but he has been a different person since his surgery.

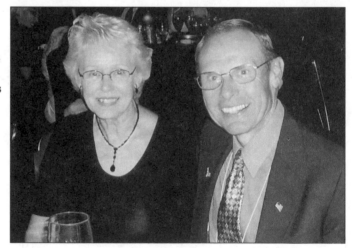

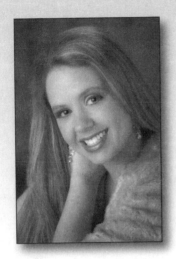

Abby Ryan

AGE: 25

HOMETOWN: La Crosse, Wisconsin

MEDICAL SITUATION:
A rare case of ulcerative colitis during infancy robs a young girl of her childhood and leads to a host of challenges—medical and social—that are finally turned around after ileostomy surgery at age eleven.

Ask most women to think back on their childhood, and they'll likely recall memories typical of little girls. They may remember slumber parties where they giggled long into the night with their favorite friends, quieting down only when someone's mother had finally had enough. They might reminisce about spending hot summer days cavorting in a swimming pool or boating on a breezy lake. Maybe they recall skipping rope on the school playground or spending quiet rainy afternoons raiding Mom's closet and dressing up like a princess.

For most women, girlhood memories are lighthearted and carefree, at least when viewed through the friendly prism of time. For others, though, childhood memories can be vastly different.

Abby Ryan falls into the latter category. Actually, Abby's earliest childhood recollections aren't even her own. "My parents can tell so many stories that I don't remember," the twenty-five-year-old third-grade schoolteacher said. She certainly doesn't recall being diagnosed with ulcerative colitis when she was only fourteen months old. Nor can she remember her large intestine being removed just before she turned four, but her parents haven't forgotten.

"Abby was born healthy, but when she was about twelve months old, I noticed blood in her diapers," said Abby's mother, Barb. The concerned mother immediately scheduled an appointment with her pediatrician, who declared there was "nothing to worry about" and "lots of babies have to push hard to get the stool out."

The trouble was that Abby's stools were loose and watery—not firm and difficult to eliminate. In fact, the diarrhea-like movements happened so often that Barb eventually stopped changing her baby on a changing table. "I would stand her up in the tub and rinse her off after each diaper change," she explained.

The frequent "stooling," as her parents put it, took its toll on the toddler. Her father, Ed, recalls a time when they were in a store and he noticed Abby's energy wilt. Suddenly, she went limp. "We rushed her to the car and sped through town to the hospital," he said. "We thought she was dying." It turned out that Abby's potassium level was extremely low due to the excessive diarrhea.

Barb remembers another afternoon when Abby, not quite eighteen months old, crawled behind an old living room chair and just curled up on the floor. "She had gone to the bathroom so much that day that she was just *done*."

By now Barb had seen enough. She called the family clinic in tears and pleaded with the nurse for advice. In August 1984, Abby was admitted to a local hospital in their hometown of La Crosse, Wisconsin, for a series of tests. Nine days later, the doctors said they had found an "abnormality" in Abby's upper gastrointestinal tract. They suspected ulcerative colitis but had never seen this disease in a child so young. To confirm their suspicions, they referred the Ryans to the renowned Mayo Clinic seventy miles away in Rochester, Minnesota. After more sophisticated tests and biopsies at one of the premier health facilities in the country, the initial diagnosis was confirmed in March 1985. So began the "roller coaster" life that would outline Abby's childhood.

The Ryans had never even heard of ulcerative colitis. To help process all the new information, Barb documented everything. She would ultimately fill seven notebooks with detailed records of hospital visits, lab procedures, tests, names and amounts of drugs, along with side effects, records of improvement, and documentation of setbacks. "I just kept writing," Barb said, referring to her comprehensive account of Abby's early years, which belongs in a medical library somewhere, not in a parent's closet.

Barb's journal recorded a series of "bad flare ups" between December 1985 and February 1987. Each flare-up necessitated another trip to Rochester and the requisite invasive tests. "Abby was a real trooper," Ed said, "but it was hard on her. They were always doing rectal scopes or drawing blood, and her arms were black and blue from all the attempts to find a vein." Early in 1987, several months shy of her fourth birthday, Abby's condition worsened significantly.

"In February, she had a bad flare-up, so we took her back to Mayo," explained Barb. "Our doctor had been discussing the possibility of surgery but was hoping to avoid it. On that day, however, he said the colon had to go."

The surgeon wanted to perform what is called an ileoanal anastomosis, a procedure in which the lower portion of Abby's small intestine would be shaped into an internal pouch (a J-pouch), which would later be attached to her anal canal. The surgery would be done in two phases. The first would involve removing Abby's colon and creating the internal pouch. She would be given a temporary ileostomy at the same time, which would allow the pouch to heal. Six weeks later, she would return for the second part of the operation, where the surgeon would re-attach the new pouch to the remaining rectum and close up the ileostomy, thus restoring normal continence.

The doctors who operated on the four-year-old said her colon looked like the diseased intestine of someone who'd been suffering from colitis for years. She spent the next ten days recovering while Barb camped out at the hospital and Ed commuted back and forth every other day.

The day before Abby was scheduled to go home, however, complications set in, and the preschooler unexpectedly and explosively vomited all over her hospital bed. X-rays revealed a total, 100 percent bowel obstruction, a potentially life-threatening emergency that required immediate surgery.

"It was like starting all over," said Barb of the setback. "Although Abby had a new ileostomy to deal with, we all knew she still needed to come back for her follow-up surgery six weeks later."

So Many Unpleasant Procedures

When Abby was finally released from the hospital and allowed to recover at home, Barb learned not only how to manage Abby's stoma but also how to perform anal dilatation in preparation for the next phase of Abby's surgical procedures. The onerous duty involved inserting a gloved index finger into Abby's rectum to maintain the sphincter muscle's flexibility.

"The new pouch is attached to the rectal muscle," said Barb, explaining the need for manual dilation of Abby's sphincter muscle. "In order for the pouch to function effectively, this muscle needed to stay open. Since Abby was not eliminating rectally during the healing process, the muscle could easily close up from lack of use, which might cause a lot of trouble later."

No drugs were given to relax Abby during this unpleasant procedure, which needed to be done twice a day for six weeks. Though it was hard on little Abby in the beginning—Barb says her preschooler "cried and cried" at first—Abby eventually found a way to cope. She would say to her father, "OK, Dad, come and hold my hand." Ed would stand beside his daughter and take her tiny hand into his. She in turn would look up into his eyes, squeeze his hand tightly, and tell him she was going to be "super brave."

On May 13, 1987—almost two months after the initial surgery to remove her colon and six weeks after life-saving bowel obstruction surgery—Abby returned to the Mayo Clinic to be "reconnected," as Ed and Barb put it. According to Ed, Abby was among the youngest, if not the youngest, person in the United States to undergo this procedure. Not the sort of record that parents would want to see their child capture.

Unfortunately, this was not the end of Abby's story. There was a brief respite—maybe four or five months—when it appeared as if the J-pouch was functioning properly, but then the pouch became infected, not an uncommon surgical complication.

"We went from colitis to pouchitis," said Barb. "For the next six years, we dealt with the exact same kinds of symptoms we faced *before* Abby's surgery, as well as the same futile attempts to manage those symptoms. We're talking Imodium. Antibiotics. Metamucil. Enemas. Prednisone. Nighttime diapers. Dehydration. IV treatments . . . we dealt with them all."

Abby said she felt like she was a guinea pig for every new medication that came down the pike. "Some would work for a few weeks, and then I'd get sick again. And because I didn't have a large intestine, I found it very hard to stay hydrated, especially during the hot and humid summer months. I'd frequently end up in the hospital for a couple for days just to get re-hydrated. I was in so often that the nurses on the pediatric floor got to know me personally. They'd put me in my favorite room and start the IV while I'd watch my favorite movie and get 're-booted,' so to speak. It was almost like a little vacation." As if a hospital visit can ever be compared to taking some time off from life.

"Abby seemed to know when it was time to go in for a treatment," added Barb. "One time at the hospital, she crawled into my lap and said, 'I'm so glad we're here, Mom, because I know this IV will make me feel better.' That's not to say she wasn't afraid. Who likes to be poked all the time? But she was a real trooper. Whenever we had to go in for a treatment, she would say she was going to be 'super brave.' But I do remember once when she was about eight years old and she didn't want to go. She said, 'I can't be super brave no more, Mom.' That was the one time I couldn't handle it anymore and finally broke down crying."

When Abby was seven, her parents started taking her to a facility closer to home in Madison, Wisconsin. There her new doctor immediately prescribed between thirty and forty milligrams of prednisone every other day. The aggressive treatment seemed to alleviate the symptoms but brought on some other challenges.

By the time Abby entered second grade, the side effects from the powerful drug were evident. She had gained weight ("Her cheeks were like a chipmunk," said Barb) and spider angiomas and sores adorned her face. In addition, the prednisone treatment was affecting Abby's growth. She fell way behind other children in her age group. Whenever the doctor tried to wean her off the powerful medication, however, her symptoms returned with a vengeance. "This was the roller coaster we lived on for several years," explained Barb. "Back and forth to the hospital in Madison, more drugs, terrible side effects."

Meanwhile, life at school was rough. Though her parents had done a great job advocating for Abby by speaking to teachers individually and making sure their daughter's needs were being met, Abby still found herself the object of taunts and teasing. "Kids made fun of me, especially when I was on high doses of prednisone. They'd call me 'Fatso' and say I couldn't play with them. At recess, I'd stand beside the teacher. When she asked me why I didn't play with my friends, I'd say, 'I don't want to play with them. I want to stand with you.' " If she did befriend another child, she typically chose another outcast like herself—the obese girl, the hyperactive boy, the goofy kid with a Mohawk.

Abby couldn't help but feel as if the other kids resented her because she had "special" privileges, and this complicated her predicament even more. "On the one hand, I didn't want to be perceived as the 'goody-two-shoes, suck-up girl' who stood next to the teacher at recess and never needed a bathroom pass," she said.

"But, on the other hand, I *had* to be that person because of how sick I was."

Abby often came home from school and flopped down on the couch, physically and emotionally exhausted. "I just figured kids were mean because they didn't understand. I knew this was something I had to deal with, so I just dealt with it as best I could."

Conflicting Routes

In 1995, when Abby was eleven, the Ryans found themselves at a crossroads. By then, they were still seeing their personal doctor in nearby Madison, but they were also consulting with physicians at the Mayo Clinic in Rochester. Specialists at each facility recommended different courses of action. Their family doctor in Madison, concerned about Abby's delayed growth and aware that puberty was just around the corner, recommended growth hormone treatments in conjunction with high doses of prednisone. He also wanted to include Abby in a research study that examined the effects of prednisone on ulcerative colitis patients. He believed that Abby, being so young, would be an excellent candidate for the study.

Of course, there were downsides. Barb would have to administer the painful growth hormone injections in Abby's upper thigh, and there was a slight risk of Abby developing cancer later on. In spite of the risks, though, the doctor felt this was the best course of action—not to mention the added benefit that Abby would be contributing to an important research study.

It was a tempting option, and if the Ryans had not also been consulting with doctors at the Mayo Clinic, it's a path they might have taken. But their specialist in Rochester had another idea and his own compelling reasons for her parents to consider.

After examining Abby and sending her back to the waiting room, he spoke gently but firmly to Barb. "This little girl's quality of life is so low," he said. "You could argue that she doesn't even have a life. She needs ileostomy surgery, and she needs it now."

Barb and Ed knew intuitively that he was right, but they agonized over the decision. "One doctor was saying that ostomy surgery would restore Abby's quality of life," said Ed. "The other was telling us that we should absolutely not opt for the surgery, and he even implied that we would regret making such a monumental decision for a child so young."

Ed and Barb talked late into the night, examining the pros and the cons of each option. Barb says she tossed and turned, but by the time she woke up early the next morning, she felt she knew what had to be done. When they informed Abby about the decision, the eleven-year-old went ballistic, begging her parents not to put her through another painful and demanding surgery.

"I cried and cried," Abby remembers. "I did all the things that kids do to try to convince their parents to change their mind. I promised I wouldn't be bad anymore. I told them they wouldn't have to pay me an allowance. I begged them let me try something else . . . anything else. But, at the end of the day, I was too young and unable to dissuade my parents. When they explained their rationale to me, they explained that the biggest issue really came down to their desire for me to have a better quality of life."

In February 1994, Abby took time off from the fifth grade and returned to Rochester for ileostomy surgery. "After I woke up, I immediately felt different," she recalled. "I felt like this was the start of something good." Indeed, when Abby describes those first months after her surgery today, it's as if she's describing a bird set free from a cage. "I could walk through a department store and not be fearful of having an accident. I could drive to Grandma's without having to pull over every half hour to use the bathroom . . . it was *fantastic!*"

A month after surgery, Abby was a different child. Now that her body was absorbing the nutrients that it had been losing all those years, she blossomed . . . and started to grow. Her parents noticed the physical differences almost immediately. "I remember looking at her one day and admiring how nice and full her legs and arms looked," said Barb. "Just like a regular kid."

Her dad agrees. "For six years she had been trapped in a pouch-infected, prednisone-bloated body that couldn't do anything. Once she got her energy back, there was no stopping her. She developed a can-do attitude in which she felt there was nothing she *couldn't* do."

When Abby got to middle school, she joined the choir, took up the alto sax, and tried out for the softball and basketball teams. By the time she reached high school, she added show choir and drama to the mix. In her junior year, she was voted to the prom court, and in her senior year, she was elected homecoming princess by her fellow classmates! It was clear that she had come a long way in a short amount of time and seemed to be making up for all of the lost years.

Still a Secret, Though

Although she made tons of friends and became more outgoing, Abby never felt quite comfortable telling anyone at school about her ostomy, an inclination based largely upon the advice of a middle school counselor who cautioned her that children could be very cruel. As a result of this advice, Abby kept her ostomy a secret throughout middle school and high school—until something happened near the end of her senior year.

During a spring concert, she sang a solo. Afterwards, a woman from the audience approached the pretty and talented teenager and asked if she would consider becoming a contestant in the upcoming Miss La Crosse/Oktoberfest Pageant, a part of the Miss America Organization. Abby was flattered, but hesitant. She knew that contestants would be judged in four areas: evening gown, talent, interview, and swimsuit. It was the swimsuit part that terrified her. "I never liked being seen in a bathing suit on the beach," she admitted. But she thought about it long and hard and decided to give it a try.

At the first practice session, contestants were asked to select a platform—a cause or issue they believed in passionately, and for which they would become an advocate. Abby couldn't help but reflect on her childhood: the years in and out of hospitals fighting dehydration and infection while wrestling with her inflammatory bowel disease. The summers spent indoors while other kids played outside. The sleepovers she missed because she feared nighttime accidents. She could still feel the sting of rejection from being teased and bullied in the schoolyard. She recalled how she longed to be accepted for who she was but was instead shunned because of a disease she could not control. Then she reflected on how ileostomy surgery had, in a sense, restored her childhood. That's when she *knew* she had found her platform . . . a real platform she could speak passionately about.

Her courage was rewarded on September 15, 2001, when eighteen-year-old Abby Ryan was crowned Miss La Crosse/Oktoberfest. For the swimsuit competition, she wore a "tasteful, one-piece blue suit," as she described it, and her platform was "You Are Not Alone: Crohn's and Colitis Awareness." It was the same platform she would use in many subsequent pageants.

In 2002, she vied for the Miss Wisconsin title while wearing a stylish, hot-pink, *two-piece* swimsuit and finished among the Top Ten. Since then, she has been crowned Miss Western Wisconsin 2004, Miss Midwest 2006, and Miss Mississippi Valley 2007.

When she was twenty-four years old in June 2007, she decided to compete a second time for the Miss Wisconsin title. Having reached the age limit for competing in the Miss America pageants and knowing this would be her last shot at becoming the only Miss America contestant to ever compete with an ostomy, she decided to go out in style by selecting the skimpiest swimsuit her physical condition would allow.

"I was in the best shape of my life," she said, pointing out that most young women ostomates dread the idea of revealing so much skin in public. "I felt confident and comfortable, so I pushed the envelope and wound up making the Top Ten in that pageant. Even better, I won the Spirit of Miss America Award, an award that is voted on by the contestants themselves. It was an amazing honor and something that really touched me."

Despite her success in beauty pageants, Abby's story doesn't have a fairy-tale ending, though, at least not the way Hollywood would write it.

Her health problems have not gone away. She nearly lost her life two years ago during a routine anal dilatation procedure. Recently, her ulcerative colitis diagnosis was changed to Crohn's disease, and she continues to suffer from the residual effects of pouchitis because the doctors were unable to remove the infected pouch at the time of her ileostomy surgery. The pouch has since adhered to her female organs and remains lodged inside her to this day, unnecessary and superfluous, but still causing problems. There is some concern that the pouch may create additional issues should she decide to have children. So, for Abby, the battle continues, but it is a battle that is ever-so fulfilling.

Despite all of this, Abby remains a tireless advocate for Crohn's and Colitis Awareness, speaking publicly at local and national events, raising funds by participating in Walk-a-Thons and Bowl-a-Thons, serving as a counselor at United Ostomy Association Youth Camps, and—on a more personal level—quietly influencing the children in her elementary school classroom in La Crosse.

"I talk with my third-grade students about what it was like to be teased when I was a little girl and about how much it hurt," said the first-year teacher, who often invites her young students to sit in a circle during class to talk about things like teasing and bullying.

"They're very surprised when they find out that I've won beauty pageants and that even people like their teacher, Miss Ryan, got bullied," she said. "It's so important for children to know how their actions at this age can affect people for the rest of their lives."

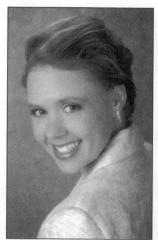

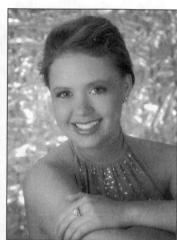

Beauty queen Abby Ryan has won numerous beauty pageants and was even willing to compete in a two-piece bathing suit—following ostomy surgery—in front of the judges and the public.

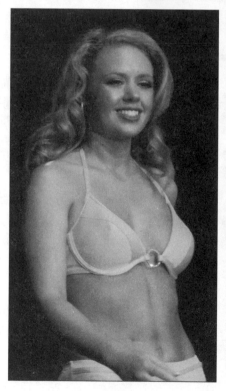

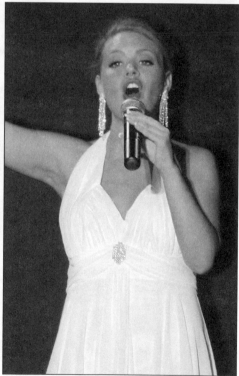

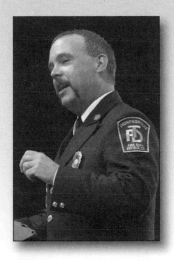

Scott Ellis

AGE: 37

HOMETOWN: Enfield, Connecticut

MEDICAL SITUATION:
A childhood case of ulcerative colitis leads to failed "J-pouch" surgery at fifteen, followed by permanent ostomy surgery at nineteen, but doesn't prevent a young man from pursuing his dream of becoming a firefighter.

S cott Ellis considers himself a lucky guy. Though he was officially diagnosed with ulcerative colitis when he was a child, he was "lucky" that his pediatrician sent him to a specialist almost immediately. Within months of the first symptoms, his disease was "squared away, diagnosed, and treated," he remembers.

Yes, treatment for the next six years did include some powerful drugs like prednisone and sulfasalazine, but he was "lucky" the doses were apparently low enough not to produce some of the disagreeable side effects often associated with these potent drugs. And though he did have the occasional flare-up during those early years, for the most part the events were mild, and medications kept things manageable.

"It was nothing dramatic—maybe some cramping or diarrhea where I'd have to get to the bathroom fast. When those episodes persisted, my doctor would up the dosages a bit and get things back under control," Scott explained.

Scott said his luck ran out the summer before his sophomore year in high school. He had such a significant flare-up that he wound up in the hospital for two months on "complete bowel rest," only to be advised near the end of his stay that things weren't improving and that surgery would be necessary.

The doctor assured him that he was a good candidate for a new procedure called an ileoanal pull-through, more commonly known as J-pouch surgery. With few options left, Scott agreed to the surgery, but things quickly went sideways for Scott as his newly constructed pouch became infected. In fact, he would spend the next four years dealing with complications related to pouchitis.

"But I couldn't have been luckier," he said, referring to the fact that the physician assigned to his case was a nationally renowned proctologist, Dr. David Walters. "Medical students come from around the world to intern with this doctor, and suddenly he was my personal surgeon. He actually dropped the central line in my subclavian vein when they needed to extend my bowel rest for another month. That's normally a menial, first-year resident type of task, but he did it himself. I felt good about that."

And even though there were a few "bumps in the road" (his words) en route to a full recovery—including a rock-strewn detour leading to a permanent ostomy at age nineteen—Scott Ellis still believes he got off easy. "I've heard so many horror stories," remarked the thirty-seven-year-old Connecticut firefighter. "For some people, just as they get their chin up, something comes along and knocks them down again. For me, the medical part of my story from start to finish doesn't last a huge amount of time. There was only a six-year period when I was dealing with ulcerative colitis, and then I went into the surgical corrections for maybe another four-year period. Other than a few blockages over the years, I've been cruising ever since."

Most people wouldn't look back on an adolescence characterized primarily by chronic diarrhea and cramping, steroids, and several major abdominal surgeries with such equanimity. But Scott seems to take the whole experience in stride—at least outwardly. He does concede there were some internal struggles that he has only recently begun to confront, and he credits the Great Comebacks program for providing him a vehicle to deal with those. Nevertheless, when he looks back on his journey, he barely notices the potholes in the road. All he sees are milestones.

The Early Years

The fourth and youngest child of Donald and Sally Ellis, Scott was born in the summer of 1971 and grew up in Enfield, Connecticut, a small suburb outside Hartford. Other than a brief stint working as a firefighter in a neighboring city, Scott has lived in Enfield his entire life, as have his older brother and sisters, Donny, Debbie, and Lisa.

Indeed, all four siblings bought homes on the southern side of town near their parents' house. Scott jokes that "we can do a loop between all our houses in five minutes." Though Scott's older siblings are a year apart, Scott arrived on the scene some ten years after Lisa. By the time he began to exhibit symptoms of ulcerative colitis, Donny and Debbie had already moved out of the house, and Lisa—in college at the time—was only home on the weekends.

Strangely enough, Lisa also suffered from ulcerative colitis, and she herself had ostomy surgery at age twenty-five—two months after Scott had his J-pouch operation at age fifteen. Not surprisingly, Lisa's memories of Scott's early years are inextricably intertwined with her own.

"I was very aware of all of his problems since they were the same as mine," said Lisa, who is also five years removed from rectal cancer. "Both of us were always using the bathroom, and since our house only had one toilet, things could get pretty interesting. Fortunately there were only two of us kids left at home when Scott started getting sick. When he had his surgery, I wasn't living at home. I remember being on vacation in Virginia and driving overnight to make sure I saw him before his big operation. But I don't think I knew how serious it was, and my parents never let on. Our family isn't very demonstrative. We tend to just go with the flow and not ask a lot of questions."

Perhaps for similar reasons, Scott, too, tends to gloss over those early years leading up to the crisis that put him in the hospital the summer before his sophomore year. "My mother never allowed us kids to wallow in self-pity, and there was no leeway for throwing up your hands and feeling sorry for yourself," he explained. "I remember I missed most of my sophomore year because of this illness, and at one point I decided I wanted to quit school. I was worn out and had had enough. But my mom is just as stubborn as me—it's her Irish nature—and she wasn't about to let that happen.

Agreeing that her son could indeed be obstinate, Sally Ellis remembered that Scott sometimes didn't want to do things that were to his benefit, like going to school. "I think he was frustrated and probably depressed. Maybe he was also going through a teenage rebellious stage and was trying to get back at me for something," she mused. "All I knew was that he had to have at *least* a high school diploma."

Sally remembers going straight to the school counselor and informing her in no uncertain terms that Scott was going to finish high school "if I have to chase him down and make him graduate myself." The counselor, not wanting to incur the wrath of this strong-willed woman, immediately set up Scott with a tutor.

To this day Scott credits this private instructor for convincing him to not only finish his sophomore year but ultimately graduate from high school. Looking back nearly twenty years, he now sees this incident in his life as one of several significant milestones.

First of all, he realizes that the emotional turmoil he was going through at the time had a lot to do with adolescent immaturity magnified by a fear of the unknown. "My illness was wearing me down, and I couldn't fully understand all that I was dealing with," he said, recalling that pivotal year when he was ready to call it quits. "In reality, I knew I had my whole life ahead of me, but I was scared to death of surgery and, from my limited perspective, I didn't know if I could handle it all.

"I also knew I wanted to be a firefighter, but there was this nagging fear and doubt that things might not work out and I might not be able to cut it. At the time, with everything else going on, school seemed impossible. I was ready to throw in the towel. Thankfully, my mother had a better understanding of all this and pushed me to finish and graduate."

Even though she wasn't around much at that point, Lisa also remembers quite a bit of tension between Scott and his parents. "Looking back now, I think my brother blamed my parents for his problems because they had given the go-ahead for the J-pouch surgery in the first place," she said. "And when the pouch didn't work, that's when he became really angry, and he lashed out at everyone. I remember coming home from college and he seemed so defeated—his life was governed by what happened in the bathroom. It was definitely a taxing time for our family."

Scott agrees he wasn't any fun to be around, but he speculates that part of his hostility can be traced to the huge disappointment he felt when the anticipated cure of the J-pouch surgery didn't transpire.

"I'd been dealing with this illness for as long as I could remember, though for most of the time it was pretty manageable," he explained. "That last flare-up the summer before my sophomore year, however, was pretty intense. The episode came on me very suddenly and just couldn't be controlled by any medications. I found out later, after they did the pathology on my colon, that I was hours, maybe a day, away from the whole thing perforating. What a horrible time. I had been in the hospital for several weeks, and I was on IV meds, steroids, and complete bowel rest. My weight had dropped to about eighty pounds, and I was getting progressively worse with no end in sight."

Scott remembers Dr. Walters coming into his room and saying they could surgically correct things. "At the time, they were starting to do the pull-through pouch procedures, and that was what he recommended for me," Scott said. "He tried to explain exactly what was involved, but I had no idea what he was talking about. I was pretty out of it and just nodded my head and said, 'Yep, sounds good,' but in reality, I didn't have a clue. All I heard was, 'This will get better,' and that's all I needed to know. Give me a bottle of whisky and a dull butcher knife, I didn't care—I just wanted to stop hurting.

"I actually looked forward to surgery because Dr. Walters was assuring me that the pain and the stomach problems would stop. But then he explained that people with ulcerative colitis *tend* to adjust well to this type of surgery, and that nine times out of ten there will be no complications. I remember thinking, *Uh, oh*. You see, I'm usually not good with odds, which is why I don't like to gamble. If there's a 90 percent chance that everything's going to be perfect I usually fall into that 10 percent where it isn't!"

In Scott's case, the longer odds proved to be against him. After his initial surgery, he received a temporary ostomy to give him time to heal before returning for the follow-up operation to connect his internal pouch to his rectum.

In the interim months, Scott began to feel optimistic. He was eating again, gaining weight, getting stronger, and he was even putting in some work hours at a dairy farm about a mile and a half from his home. By the time he returned to the hospital for the follow-up surgery, he had regained a more positive outlook on life.

Unfortunately for Scott, there were problems with the pouch almost from the moment it was reconnected. "Basically what happened is that the pouch itself became diseased," Scott explained. "They called it pouchitis. When I first heard that word, I couldn't believe that was the technical term. I even ribbed the doctor, saying, 'You couldn't come up with a name for this condition that has a few more syllables . . . maybe a little Latin? But *pouchitis*? Jeez."

Without going into specifics, all Scott will say about the

remaining months of his sophomore year and the following summer is that they were "a nightmare." When the family sat down with Dr. Walters to discuss their options, Scott told them things had been ten times better for him when he had had the temporary ileostomy. "I was able to do everything I wanted to do," he explained. "I had gotten my weight back, was without pain, and had felt healthy for the first time in a long time. But when I got the pouch, the cramping and diarrhea, the pain and the weight loss—it all returned with a vengeance."

Dr. Walters admitted that the pouch wasn't working and agreed with Scott that he would probably be better off if they reversed the procedure and gave him a permanent ostomy. Scott and his parents felt the same way. So, at age of nineteen, Scott went under the knife one more time and left the operating bay with a permanent ostomy.

Another Milestone

By all accounts, Scott was a different person after his surgery. It was as if he had passed another important milestone in his life. His father, Donald, said that being hospitalized for so long was difficult for Scott, and that he had felt a little sorry for himself. "But once he recovered from the surgery, he seemed to become a new man. He got involved almost immediately in the fire service, and this more than anything helped him to overcome his feelings of self-pity."

Scott's sister Lisa agrees. "It's always been Scott's dream to help people, but for a while it seemed this illness was going to interfere with that dream," she said. "By the time he got his permanent ostomy, I think he realized he could live with it and that now he could be healthy and do what he really wanted to do."

What Scott wanted to do was follow in the footsteps of nearly every male member of his family. Scott is not joking when he says he had wanted to be a fireman ever since he was two years old. "I come from a family of firefighters," he said, citing a list of relatives that spans several generations and even includes a few in-laws. "When I first met my wife, Marla, I thought I'd met a 'normal' person—no firefighting background, nothing," he said, laughing. "But after we'd been dating a few months, I learned several of her uncles are retired firefighters! It's definitely in the blood on both sides of our family."

Not everyone, however, felt Scott should pursue a career in fire prevention. Lisa, in particular, had her reservations, but not because she thought Scott couldn't handle the rigors of the profession. "I knew the ostomy itself wouldn't stop him," said Lisa. "I was more worried about the fact that Scott had never wanted to discuss anything related to his surgery. He always kept it to himself and I knew that he wouldn't be able to keep it a secret at the station. I fought with him for a long time about being more open. Even when I tried to give him some sisterly advice about trying different appliances and products, he refused to engage me. I told him unless you can get comfortable talking about this, how do you think you can function in a firehouse? Firemen can be your best buddies or your worst enemies . . . but there are surely no secrets."

Learning to be more open and feeling comfortable talking about his ostomy was, in fact, one of the big milestones Scott mentions when he reflects upon his journey. "So much of my emotional growth had to do with understanding that fears are so often far worse than reality," Scott points out. "I had to learn that."

"After I passed the written exams and the physical agilities and reached the point where I was a legitimate candidate for a position in the fire department, I became concerned that my ostomy would be an issue. Of course, legally, there's no reason they couldn't hire me based on the ostomy alone. I knew intellectually that as long as a candidate meets or exceeds their standards, the department couldn't discriminate. But I still had this fear.

"I went in to my first pre-employment physical prepared with all sorts of research and was determined to fight back if they gave me a hard time. But the whole thing turned out to be pretty anti-climactic, and a big confrontation never happened. The doctor who examined me briefly commented on my ostomy and asked if it gave me any problems, and that was about it. No big deal. All that worrying for nothing. It was a big lesson and something I am reminded of all of the time."

Scott had a similar experience in the early days of his relationship with Marla before they were married. He admits to dreading what she would think of him once she learned about his ostomy. "You imagine the worst and convince yourself in your mind that there's no way you can have an intimate relationship with someone when you have an ostomy," he says smiling.

Once again, however, Scott discovered that his fears were misplaced. "Looking back, having known my wife for so many years now, I'm ashamed that I ever thought something like this would bother her," said Scott, who just marked his tenth anniversary with Marla. "She's not the kind of person to let something so superficial bother her."

Unfortunately for her, Scott said, he wasn't as secure as she was, and he carried his self-esteem issues into the marriage. "Marla was desperate to understand and help and wanted to be part of something that was such a huge part of my life," he explained, "but initially I didn't want to talk about anything related to my ostomy. It's a typical guy thing I guess—*I can deal with this myself, I don't need any help, if I don't talk about it, maybe it will go away* . . . that sort of thing. Obviously, that wasn't true, and when I finally began to open up, it became a huge turning point for me . . . and for the both of us."

Scott credits Marla for nudging him past one more milestone in his journey—telling the guys he worked with in the firehouse about his ostomy. "Up until five years ago, no one at the station knew about it," said Scott, who drives the engine for his crew and is also the rescue swimmer when the squad is needed for water emergencies.

"As I started to get a little older, I guess I began to become more comfortable with myself and also wondered what would happen if I got hurt or incapacitated on the job. I realized these are the guys who are going to keep me alive, and they needed to know what I have. Of course, Marla had been telling me this for years. She said I needed to give people a chance. Turns out she was right."

Once again, Scott discovered that the fear of the unknown was far worse than reality. "You really can't keep many secrets in a firehouse because you spend so much time together. And I knew all their secrets—their heart diseases, their cancers, their conflicts at home. One day it dawned on me, *What's the big deal if they know what I've been through?* I'd convinced myself that I had been keeping my ostomy a secret because I didn't want the guys to feel they needed to 'protect' me. But, in reality, deep down, I was scared about what they might think of me.

"Remember, we're talking about a firehouse here. A place that is run like a good ol' boys club with—how shall I put it—plenty of bathroom humor. But once again, my fears were totally blown out of proportion. A few of the guys said they knew someone who had an ostomy; others were curious and wanted to know more about what the surgeries entailed, and of course, some gave me a hard time. But ribbing comes with the territory. I can handle it."

Growing as a Person

Scott's willingness to talk freely about his ostomy and shrug off the good-natured ribbing from his fellow firemen were clear indicators to his family that he fully accepted his ostomy surgery. But it was applying for the Great Comebacks award itself that epitomized just how far Scott had grown.

"It all kind of snowballed after I started doing research on the Internet trying to learn more about ostomies, support groups, and the different products out there. I'd been wearing the same appliance since I was sixteen, always figuring that if it 'ain't broke, don't fix it,' but I was still wondering if there might be something better out there. In looking into things, I stumbled on to the Great Comebacks website and really appreciated the inspirational stories. I never thought much about sending mine in, though. To be honest, I filled out an application so I could get on some more mailing lists," Scott confessed sheepishly.

"Then, lo and behold, about a month later, Rolf Benirschke called my house and told me I had been selected as the 2007 Great Comebacks Eastern Regional Award winner! [Scott would go on to be named the 2007 National Great Comebacks Award winner.] This is embarrassing, don't tell him, but I had absolutely no idea who he was! The guys at work harassed me to no end because they're huge football fans and knew him right away. They could rattle off Rolf's stats like Dustin Hoffman in *Rain Man*. But I was just ten years old when Rolf was kicking for the San Diego Chargers, so I had no clue!"

Winning the Great Comebacks award has had a profound influence on Scott, at least in the eyes of his sister. "I was so proud of him when he won, but what made me the happiest was that he was finally willing to open up and talk about it with complete honesty," said Lisa, who admits her family had been urging her to apply for the award, too. "Keeping his ostomy a secret was always a burden on Scott, but winning the Great Comebacks award was a gift. The recognition made him more aware of the many people out there who are just like him. Since Scott's whole mission in life is to help others, this award has freed him to help people on a deeply personal level."

Scott doesn't disagree, but he takes it one step further. "Winning these awards is a huge responsibility. I have to step up and be willing to talk about my ostomy, even if I'm still uncomfortable about some things," he said. "And though I don't feel I'm different from anyone else who has experienced this kind of surgery, maybe by telling my story I can help other people who are struggling with a self-imposed reluctance to discuss it."

When asked to reflect what he's learned on this journey, Scott had a quick reply. "I've learned that I can't hate this ostomy. Yes, it upsets you, and yes, you get frustrated at times. But you can't hate it. That's something my wife, Marla, reminds me all the time. This ostomy saved my life . . . if I didn't have it, I wouldn't be here. And neither would our special children. She's right, of course. For some of us, it comes down to a choice: we either die, or we have this ostomy and we continue living with a chance to pursue our dreams. I'll take living with an ostomy any day."

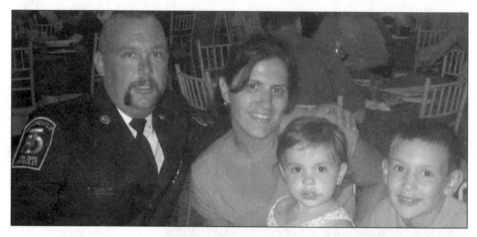

Scott Ellis and his wife, Marla, with their two children, Kaylene (3) and Matthew (9). All Scott ever wanted to do was to become a firefighter in his hometown of Enfield, Connecticut.

His dreams were almost shattered when he was forced to undergo ostomy surgery.

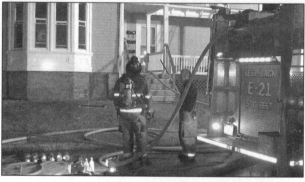

Rolf Benirschke presented Scott with the National Great Comebacks Award in 2007.

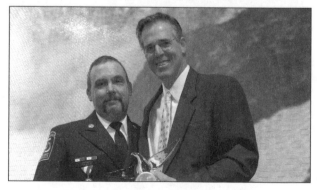

FLYING THROUGH THE TURBULENCE

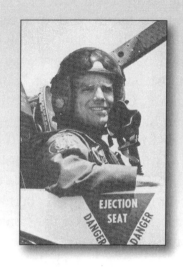

George Vogt

AGE: 53

HOMETOWN: Montgomery, Alabama

MEDICAL SITUATION:
An Air Force fighter pilot battles ulcerative colitis that threatens to ground his military career, but ostomy surgery returns him to the pilot's seat.

H *is "office" hurtles skyward, reaching 40,000 feet and withstanding up to nine times the force of gravity. He tenses his muscles against a velocity of thirteen hundred miles per hour and G-forces that would debilitate the untrained person in seconds. Yet enclosed beneath his bubble canopy, an oxygen mask concealing his expression, the fighter pilot barely suppresses the urge to laugh out loud. How many times has he done this, but each time now he can't help giggling like a schoolgirl? Flying into the wild blue yonder never gets old!*

George Vogt was raised in a close-knit military family, the youngest of three children whose parents met during World War II when George's father, Eric Vogt, was wounded on a beach landing in the South Pacific. Sent to Letterman Hospital in San Francisco for removal of shrapnel, Eric was tended to by a pretty occupational therapist named Elizabeth ("Lil") Cooper. As George's dad liked to say, "I was in bed when I met my wife!"

Eric and Lil married in 1949 and lived in the San Francisco area before being transferred to Hawaii in 1963, where Lieutenant Colonel Vogt would be stationed for the duration of the Vietnam conflict. Young George was eight, middle sister Libbie was eleven, and oldest brother Eric was thirteen when the family settled on the island of Oahu in the secluded beach community of Kailua, twelve miles northeast of Honolulu. Surrounded by the powdery white beaches, translucent seas, and sweet-scented blossoms one typically associates with a tropical paradise, George balanced his time between sports, school, and—when he could sneak away— surfing. The windward side of the island supplied the postcard-perfect waves, and a paucity of tourists provided ample elbowroom for the locals to enjoy them.

The type of kid who couldn't sit still for long, George excelled in just about everything he did. "He was talented and popular," said Libbie, now a family law attorney living in Santa Barbara and one of George's most ardent admirers. Although only two-and-a-half years separate the siblings chronologically, they were four school grades apart due to a late start kindergarten (his) and a skipped grade (hers).

Perhaps because of that grade span, Libbie adopted a less sisterly, more motherly bearing. And though she regards her brother as a "tough American hero" and "a warrior with a strong, solid inner strength," she says he has a kind and gentle side, as well. "I've heard it said that if you want to know how a man is going to treat his wife, look at how he treats his mother. Until the day she died, my brother treated my mother like a queen. Even animals gravitate toward him," she added, laughing. "I could tell you a million stories about that."

She settles on just one for now—the time George tamed a ferocious Malaccan Cockatoo named Dundee while they were lunching at a swanky resort in Palm Springs, California. It's a good story and mostly true, though George does point out that Libbie has a tendency to embellish whenever she talks about him. "She'll tell you I not only flew F-16s but that I also landed one on the moon," he joked.

One of Libbie's favorite anecdotes—one she believes epitomizes her brother's personality and which even George will corroborate—hearkens back to their early childhood, when George was in kindergarten and she attended the fourth grade. "We were having dinner, and the question came up about how many players make up a football team, what each player does, and so on," Libbie began. "George insisted he could handle every position himself. Dad explained the concept of teamwork and how each player has a certain skill that contributes to the team. When that explanation didn't work, we tried reasoning with George logically—if nothing else, you can't punt the football by yourself. You need someone to hike you the ball! But George remained unconvinced. He had a self-concept that he could do anything and everything better than anyone else. It's a confident, self-assured, never-say-no attitude that almost certainly sustained him when he took ill years later."

Flying at Full Throttle

George was almost thirty years old and his career in the Air Force just beginning to peak when he developed ulcerative colitis while stationed in Korea in 1985. The virulence of the disease interrupted a career path that had taken off at full throttle after joining the Air Force six years earlier at age twenty-four. George says that he didn't know what he wanted to do straight out of college and that joining the military was almost an afterthought. Yet it's clear he was deeply influenced by his father's military career, so much so that the decision, though belated, seemed inevitable.

"I've always looked up to my dad," George said, reflecting on the decision-making process that led him to ultimately choose the military after a brief detour that included supervising a ski lift crew at Lake Tahoe for a year and then attending law school for another before finally settling on the Air Force.

"When I realized I didn't want to go into law, that's when I started thinking, *There's nothing wrong with the military. After all, Dad was an officer, and I've always wanted to fly.* I talked with my recruiters, discussed my options with friends and family, and on November 26, 1979, I raised my right hand and joined the Air Force. It was the best move I've ever made. As corny as it sounds, the military was more than a job to me—it was a calling to follow in my dad's footsteps. My eyes still mist up when I think of what he and I have in common."

After successfully attending the Flight Screening Program to determine whether he had an aptitude for flying, George proceeded on to Officer Training School and was commissioned as a Second Lieutenant on April 1, 1980. He spent a year training to be a pilot at Laughlin Air Force Base in Texas, graduated in April 1981, and remained at Laughlin for several years as a pilot instructor before his personal ambition to fly his own fighter was finally realized. He began his training in the F-16 and arrived at Kunsan Air Base in Korea in 1984. It was there his health troubles began.

George had been stationed in Korea for less than a year when he started having difficulty sleeping, became easily fatigued, and experienced frequent episodes of diarrhea and cramping. Suspecting his symptoms might be related to the new environment and an unfamiliar diet, he kept things to himself and tried to ignore what was happening. "I'm the type of person who thinks if you get sick, you just tough it out," he said. "So I worked out a little harder and hoped I'd get better in time—a wonderful, non-medical technique," he added with a laugh. "Unfortunately, it didn't help."

George distinctly remembers the day when it became clear that the macho approach wasn't working. "I was coming off what was called a Simulated Surface to Air Missile Attack," he recalled. "I was a couple thousand feet up and had pulled straight down to the ground at about seven-and-a-half to eight G's—a G-force that most people can't handle but which is fairly routine for a trained pilot. I'd never had a problem with it before, but this time everything went gray. Pilots are trained to recognize symptoms of oxygen deprivation, however, and take appropriate action before blacking out. So I rolled the airplane out and pointed it back up toward the sky and was fortunately able to finish the mission. Afterwards, a little shaken, I went directly to the flight surgeon. I think a bit of my macho, I-don't-need-to-see-a-doctor mindset was finally overcome by safety issues. Something was clearly wrong, and I knew it."

The flight surgeon considered all the triggers that could lead to chronic diarrhea, lethargy, weight loss, and fatigue, and eventually settled on ulcerative colitis as a possible culprit. "The way I understand it, this disease is a diagnosis of exclusion," George said, explaining that doctors tend to rule everything else out first before narrowing it down to colitis. To be certain of the diagnosis, the flight surgeon sent George to the 121st Evac Hospital (think "MASH") in Seoul, a four-hour bus ride down the coast, for more sophisticated testing. Test results still weren't conclusive, however, so George returned to Kunsan and was assigned desk duty and bed rest to try to settle things down. A few weeks later, the flight surgeon walked in to where George was working, took one look at him and said, "Get to the hospital—you don't look good."

And he didn't. Dehydrated and emaciated, George was immediately hooked up to IVs in the four-bed holding hospital at Kunsan before being airlifted back to the 121st Evac Hospital in what turned out to be somewhat of a harrowing journey. "It was during a snowstorm when they put me on a stretcher and rushed me out to a waiting Black Hawk helicopter," said George. "Everyone was huddled down and worried about me, but all I could think was, 'Cool! I've never ridden in one of *these* before!' "

Because of the hazardous weather conditions, the helicopter was forced to land about a half hour short of its destination. George was shuttled into a waiting ambulance for the remainder of the journey—a thrilling jaunt in its own right. "The driver drove so erratically I thought we were all going to die in the ambulance before we even got to the hospital," he remembers shaking his head.

George spent that December hovering precariously close to death, according to Libbie, who flew to Seoul the day after George called from the hospital to tell his mother he was ill. "We didn't know at the very beginning if he was going to make it or not, and we were devastated," Libbie said. "Mom called me in tears, very confused about what was happening. So I said, 'Don't worry, Mom, I'll take it from here.' I got on the phone, and it took me about twenty minutes to get through to the hospital, and a little longer before I could actually speak with George. He was very distraught and didn't know how serious the illness was—he just knew something was terribly wrong. I said, 'I'll be there within twenty-four hours.'"

And she was. After a series of phone calls and a mad dash to the airport to catch a flight, she arrived in Korea at 2:00 in the morning with a hundred dollars and her passport. After retrieving her luggage, she headed directly to the USO (United Service Organization) desk and said, "My brother's in the hospital. I have no reservations. What do I do?" Within the hour, the USO settled her in at the beautiful Sheraton Hotel in downtown Seoul, and by daybreak she was sitting beside her brother in his hospital room.

George still gets choked up thinking about the lengths his sister took to be with him that devastating December. "She totally took charge, interfacing with the doctors and nurses and doing the things family members do for loved ones who are hospitalized. I was so sick by then that they'd put me on total bowel rest and had pumped me so full of drugs I looked like a balloon."

In spite of the aggressive medical intervention, George continued to go downhill. At one point, the doctors spoke privately with Libbie and expressed concern about his failure to respond to treatment. "His lead doctor took me aside and said, 'Your brother is fading away, and we don't understand why. He seems to be especially despondent. Is there something about Christmas that we need to know about?'" Libbie recalled. "I said, 'Oh my God, that's *right*. Our father died on Christmas morning ten years ago. This Christmas will be the tenth anniversary of his death!'"

Libbie had hoped to return to the States to be with her mother for Christmas, but she agreed to stay a little longer so George wouldn't feel abandoned during this crucial time. After changing her flight and extending her reservation at the hotel, she did what most people do during the Christmas holidays—she went shopping.

"They had these fabulous little shops at the Sheraton. I bought a gorgeous bouquet of Hawaiian flowers. Then I noticed a magnificent gingerbread house on display in one of the store windows. I asked how much it cost, and the shop owner said it was for display purposes only. When I explained what was going on with my brother, she agreed to sell it to me. So on Christmas morning I arrived at the hospital, carrying a huge Hawaiian bouquet and this amazing gingerbread house," she remembers with a smile.

Running into Regulations

Whether it was the familiar fragrance of orchids and plumeria, the comforting cheer of the gingerbread house, or the dogged devotion of a loving sister—or a combination of them all—George began to feel better. Once stabilized, he was transported to Clark Air Base in the Philippines, the Air Force's regional hospital for Southeast Asia.

During his brief stay there, George spoke at length with the gastroenterologist, and for the first time he began to hear phrases like "It's incurable" and "You'll likely never fly again." The pronouncements were hard to take, but as a professional pilot, he understood the reasoning behind such decisions. Even with medication, ulcerative colitis is unpredictable, and Air Force regulations are strict regarding combat personnel. Even such seemingly insignificant health deficiencies like not having 20/20 vision require a specific waiver.

George returned stateside in February 1986 and was assigned to Travis Air Force Base in Northern California, where he supervised enlisted airmen in the surgery clinic at David Grant Medical Center while awaiting formal evaluation to determine whether or not he could remain in the Air Force. Meanwhile, he began feeling well again—so well that the doctors started tapering him off the medication he had been taking. But any illusions he harbored about a quick recovery and a return to flight status were dispelled during a visit to see his sister in Los Angeles.

"Libbie and I had gone to see a game at Dodger Stadium," he recalled. "During the drive home, I suddenly felt very tired. The food I'd eaten wasn't sitting right, and it was just all too familiar. I looked at Libbie and said, 'It's back.' The doctors resumed the higher dose of drugs to see if they could get things back under control, but this time nothing seemed to help. I felt like I was on the same path I'd been on in Korea. That's when they started talking about surgery."

The head surgeon at the base believed George would be an ideal candidate for a relatively new procedure in which his entire colon and the lining of his rectum would be removed and an internal "S" pouch would be created out of his small intestine. The procedure involved creating a temporary diverting ileostomy for two months so that the internal pouch would have time to heal.

At that point, George would return to the hospital where the ileostomy would be taken down and everything would be internalized. Though the new procedure posed some risk, George—who refers to himself as somewhat of a "Pollyanna" and who sheepishly admits that his favorite song is "Over the Rainbow"—liked the idea, mainly because he felt that by having an internal pouch it would allow him to return to as normal a life as possible. Even potential complications could be handled, "Pollyanna" reasoned, and he could always switch to an ostomy down the road, if necessary.

Once the decision to have surgery was made, the next step was selecting a surgeon. Enter Libbie once again. The Air Force surgeon who was slated to do the operation had performed only two of these new delicate procedures, so Libbie approached the head of Internal Medicine and asked for the name of the best surgeon in the country. "I told him money was not an issue. I explained that both my mother and I would mortgage our houses, if necessary, if there wasn't someone in the military who could do the operation. He tried to assure me that this doctor would be fine. But then I asked who he would want doing this surgery if it was *his* wife or child on the operating table, and that seemed to do the trick. He said, 'OK, you win. The man you want is Dr. Ted Schrock at the University of California San Francisco Medical Center.' "

The rest, as Libbie likes to say, is history. As it turned out, Dr. Schrock, who according to George "practically wrote the book on this kind of surgery," was a Naval Reserve officer who fulfilled his reserve duty by training Air Force surgeons in the very hospital where George was stationed. Dr. Schrock agreed to do the operation on the condition that the surgery take place in a military operating theater where medical school students could watch and surgical interns could take part.

"As I recall, they cancelled everything on the agenda, and I was the main attraction for that day," said George with a smile. "And because I was in a military hospital, my treatment was paid for. I think it cost me about $3.50 a day. We're talking about an operation that typically costs about a hundred grand! I have nothing but good things to say about my military medical care."

George remained in the hospital for a little over a week. His memories of those first days are vague. He remembers the stitches and the tubes, seeing an ostomy bag hanging from his side, and he remembers a lot of pain. But what he distinctly *doesn't* remember is feeling sick. "There's a big difference in my mind between feeling pain and feeling ill. I'll take pain any time over feeling sick."

George convalesced at his mother's house and gradually regained both his strength and his weight. His follow-up surgery to close the ostomy two months later was uneventful, and from that point on, it was merely a matter of getting accustomed to the internal pouch, adjusting his diet, and getting back in shape—which he did, and fast. A couple months after his grand operation, he felt well enough to go skiing. For all intents and purposes, George was back to his pre-colitis self, and he saw no reason why he couldn't return to his military career.

No Sign Off

Unfortunately, the Air Force didn't agree. About six months after George's surgery, his case was brought before two boards to determine whether he was fit to serve. The first board was the Medical Evaluation Board (MEB), which is tasked with deciding if a specific medical condition is compatible with military service. Active duty physicians not involved with a patient's case typically serve on this board. All MEB decisions are then sent to a second board, known as the Professional Evaluation Board (PEB). This group formally determines whether a patient's medical condition will preclude the patient from performing his duties.

In George's case, the MEB approved his return to military service, but the PEB overruled the decision. George was out. All that remained was to process the paperwork.

George remembers the day he stood before the clerk who informed him that he was being medically retired. "The first thing I said to him was, 'How do I appeal?' The clerk seemed flustered and said, 'I'm not sure. I guess there is an appeal process, but people don't usually appeal these decisions.' And I said, 'I'm not your usual people. I'd like to appeal.'

"My reasoning was like this: I believe each of us is the primary expert on what we can or cannot do. If we can give a realistic assessment of what we're capable of doing, then I don't think we should give up until someone either says yes or explains why no is the right answer. I can accept no if it comes with a good explanation, but when no is just no, then I'm going to say, *Who else can I ask? Who has the authority to give me a waiver? How high do I need to go to get the answer I'm looking for?*"

And so the appeal process began. Starting at the lowest echelons and wending its way up the chain of command, George's case eventually landed on the desk of the Air Force Surgeon General in the Pentagon.

It was July 1987 when the PEB reversed its decision to force George to medically retire, but because he had no colon, they would still not authorize him to fly—stating that having no colon was a significant medical liability that Air Force regulations could not overlook. In his appeal, George argued that these regulations did not apply to him because of his new internal pouch, but the military still wouldn't budge.

Not giving up, George took and passed a flight physical in August and applied for a flight waiver. In October 1987, a little over a year after his surgery, and after many letters of support from other patients who had returned to active lifestyles following this type of surgery, the waiver was finally approved, and George Vogt became the very first pilot in the history of the Air Force to be granted the right to fly without a colon! He was ecstatic and felt especially good when the Air Force decided to update its regulations to allow this kind of surgery for the future.

George admits that his long journey was discouraging at times, not knowing if he'd ever fly again, but he speaks highly of the officials who handled his case. "While it was frustrating, I found out that the system *does* work," he said, referring to the appeals process. "I am amazed at how receptive and open they were to giving me a chance. They could have easily said, 'We have enough pilots—we don't need to take a chance on this one.' But they didn't. Once they let me come back, I was determined to prove they had made the right decision. I believe I owe my career to those people who went out on a limb for me and gave me a second chance."

George is aware that his "comeback" may seem more glamorous because of his unusual profession, but he sees no difference between his comeback and that of anyone else. "There's an increased love of life, a heightened appreciation, that all of us who face this illness and have this surgery share when we come back. We feel so fortunate to be able to do the things we did before we got sick we almost can't believe it," he explained with a smile.

"Surgery doesn't change who you are. Surgery didn't make me less of a pilot. It merely allowed me to continue doing what was normal for me. I believe we make 'great comebacks' by coming back to what's normal for us. For some people, normal may be programming a computer, performing a piano concerto, or raising children. But for me, normal is when I'm flying high at 25,000 feet above sea level at nearly two times the speed of sound. There's no feeling like it—the feeling like I'm on top of the world!"

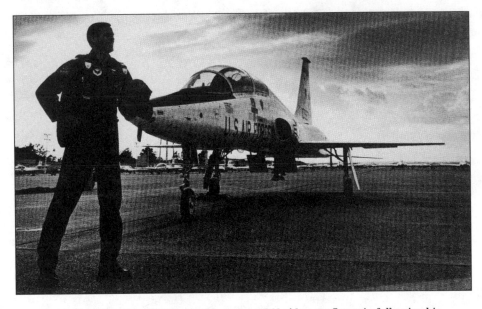

Air Force fighter pilot George Vogt was told he'd never fly again following his ostomy surgery, but through hard work, determination, and a desire to pursue his passion to fly, he was able to return to the skies.

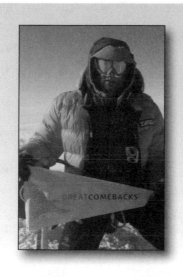

Rob Hill

AGE: 37

HOMETOWN: Vancouver, British Columbia

MEDICAL SITUATION:
A mountaineering enthusiast
overcomes Crohn's disease and
ileostomy surgery to scale the
highest mountains in the world.

Ever since Sir Edmund Hillary and his Sherpa guide, Tenzing Norgay, became the first climbers to reach the summit of Mt. Everest in 1953, nearly 2,500 others have followed their icy footsteps to the 29,029-foot summit.

Many climb the world's tallest peak for the sheer thrill—or terror, if you've read Jon Krakauer's bestselling book, *Into Thin Air*—of accomplishing a feat that few ever attempt . . . and fewer complete. They are drawn to the challenge of scaling the majestic Mt. Everest "because it's there," as British climber George Mallory famously said when asked why he would ever attempt to ascend the world's highest peak.

Climbing Mt. Everest remains one of the most dangerous undertakings confronting men and women. Despite the fact that close to 200 climbers have died in the attempt, the earth's tallest pinnacle attracts climbers of all levels, from well-experienced mountaineers to amateur novices willing to pay $75,000 for professional mountain guides to lead them to the top. Every May and September, several hundred attempt to reach the "roof of the world" during two small windows of opportunity.

Let's face it: some have attempted to scale Everest because they wanted to go into the record books as a "first." Much fanfare was made in the United States when James Whittaker became the first American to reach the summit in 1963. The first woman, Junko Tabei of Japan, arrived at the top on May 16, 1975. The first ascent without oxygen was by mountaineering legend Reinhold Messner in 1978, who two years later made the first solo ascent. Lydia Bradey of New Zealand was the first woman to reach the top without oxygen in 1988. The first married couple to summit together was Andrej and Marija Stremfelj of Slovenia in 1990, the same year Peter Hillary became the first son of a summiter to summit Everest. The first legally blind person, Erik Weihenmeyer, reached the top in 2001, and Gary Guller became the first person with only one arm to summit Everest in 2003.

On April 6, 2008, Rob Hill, a thirty-seven-year-old expert climber from British Columbia, arrived at Everest's base camp with another "first" in mind: becoming the first ostomate to reach the summit. He could truthfully say that all 2,436 men and women who climbed Everest before him had something in common: they had a colon. Rob's had been removed thirteen years earlier.

Mt. Everest would be the crowning achievement of Rob's quest to climb the "Seven Summits"—the tallest peak on each of the seven continents. When he arrived at Everest's base camp, Rob had successfully climbed:

- Mount McKinley (Denali) in North America (located in Alaska at 20,320 feet)
- Aconcagua in South America (located in the Andes mountains of Argentina at 22,841 feet)
- Vinson Massif in Antarctica (located in the Ellsworth Mountains at 16,050 feet)
- Kilimanjaro in Africa (located in Tanzania at 19,341 feet)

- Elbrus in Europe (located in the Caucasus Mountains of Russia at 18,510 feet)
- Carstensz Pyramid in Oceania (located in the Maoke Mountains of Indonesia at 16,024 feet)

The only mountain missing on his résumé was Mt. Everest, by far the most difficult of the Seven Summits, a revered peak where every climber knows the stakes are stratospherically high. At 29,029 feet, Everest is nearly as high as passenger jets at cruising altitude, and the lung-shredding atmosphere—barely one-third the pressure of sea-level air—is super cold. Temperatures are often 40 degrees below zero.

When Rob and his nine-man Canadian expedition team arrived at the 17,770-foot high Base Camp in April, they had spent more than a week trekking around the foot of Everest. The plan was to acclimatize to the altitude and bitter cold at Base Camp, and then, if everything went well, to make their assault on the Everest summit three weeks later.

Back in Seattle, a group of doctors tracked Rob's progress via the Internet, even though his digestive health had never caused him any problems on the six previous Seven Summit climbs. Meanwhile, Rob made day hikes around the Base Camp, gazing up at Everest and wondering how good it would feel to climb the world's tallest peak and complete his quest to climb the Seven Summits. That feat had been accomplished by far fewer climbers—around 200.

Of course, none of them were ostomates, either.

The First Mountain to Climb

Rob Hill was born in Kamloops, British Columbia, in 1970, the second of three children to Norman and Cheryl Hill. Dad was in the forestry industry, and Mom was an accountant. Family life revolved around the outdoors: skiing in winter and hiking in the summer. Rob started skiing when he was four years old, and by the time he entered elementary school, he was an experienced camper and an accomplished runner. He ran his first 26.2-mile marathon in the second grade—because he wanted to, not because his parents forced him. He typically ran four to eight miles each morning before school.

When he reached his teens, his father introduced him to rock climbing at the nearby peaks in the Canadian Rockies. "I really liked technical climbing from the start because of the physical and mental challenge," Rob said. "You always have to have a clear focused mind when you're climbing, and I liked that aspect since the intensity on the mountain was different than when I played team sports like soccer."

Climbing became the family sport in the Hill family. When springtime turned into longer days in the Pacific Northwest, his father would take Rob, his older brother, Don, and younger sister, Ellen, to a local outcropping after work, where he would string up ropes on a sheer face of rock. Not only did his technical climbing skills improve rapidly, but Rob showed an aptitude for finding just the right handhold and just the right route to the top.

He breezed through high school in Merritt, and then moved about 400 kilometers (250 miles) southwest to Vancouver to figure out what he wanted to do next in life. He worked a few years as a cabinetmaker and in antique restoration. Then a job opportunity—a good opportunity—became available at Motorola in the spring of 1994.

Rob was twenty-three-years old, a young man who had never been sick a day in his life except for an occasional flu bug. A couple of weeks before his job interview with Motorola, Rob ate some cream cheese that had apparently gone bad. Something went haywire in his digestive tract because that night he was hit with everything: nausea, vomiting, and diarrhea.

Even though he woke up weakened, feeling awful, and not understanding what had hit him, Rob didn't want to miss his job interview with Motorola. After all, this was a Fortune 500 company making waves in the cellular phone market, and Rob wanted to get in on the ground floor. Upon arrival at the Motorola human resources department, however, he decided he was feeling too sick to take the job interview. He asked if he could return the following day.

When Rob returned, he *still* felt horrible, but he toughed out the interview and got the job managing the shipping and receiving operation in the warehouse. His physical ills didn't improve much during the first weeks on the job, but his new boss was understanding and told him to take time off to get well. "My boss's support was tremendous," Rob said. "My medical expenses were paid for, so I knew I had a good job with a good company."

His doctor diagnosed Rob fairly quickly with Crohn's disease. "It was good to know so early because I could say to myself, 'Okay, it's Crohn's disease.' But I had no idea what Crohn's disease really was," Rob said. "I had never heard of it before. So I started researching and learning as much as I could and that really helped me deal with being so sick."

His medical team started him on drugs right away—a high dose of prednisone and other immune system blockers. "I think I was on everything out there, which helped keep me alive but never helped me go into remission," Rob said. "My symptoms would come on extremely strong and then dissipate, but they never went away. I was still going multiples times to the bathroom each day and feeling nauseated whenever I tried to eat something. This prompted my body to start surviving off my muscle mass, and I visibly weakened."

Rob was a buff guy with a muscular five-foot, eleven-inch frame before the symptoms arrived. Over the next eighteen months, his strapping physique—honed by years of rock climbing and mountaineering—lost definition and strength. His weight dipped so quickly from 185 pounds to 105 pounds that he stopped weighing himself. Rob was sure he was being punished for something. Whenever the stabbing pains ebbed, he reflected on the "Why me?" questions that reverberated through his mind.

The prednisone also did a number on his mental state. In his frustration, he lashed out at his family, and his mother remembers his short fuse. "He blew up from time to time," Cheryl said. "He had a short temper, and when talking to him his answers were short—

shorter than they needed to be."

Against this backdrop, Rob coped as best he could. Sometimes he adopted the rock climber mindset, the one that told him that he could conquer the mountain by sheer will. "I was stubborn, thinking that I would get healthy if I continued to ignore the feelings of illness, but I could never make the symptoms go away," Rob said reflectively. "After a couple of weeks running to the bathroom every thirty minutes and feeling physically ill around the clock, I realized that this wasn't something I could easily bounce back from."

A Relative Helps Out

While he was struggling to feel better, his mother's younger sister, Aunt Ida, suddenly entered the hospital to have ostomy surgery. Rob wasn't told at the time, however. "Everything was kind of hush-hush and a big secret," he said. "Then when I found out what she had gone through, I wondered: *Why would something like that be hidden in a family that was so close?*"

That was a great question. Eventually, Rob took the initiative and reached out to his aunt, who lived in Victoria, an hour-long ferry ride from Vancouver, with phone calls and occasional visits. "We would talk constantly about what she had gone through, and any time I had a question, she was always very helpful," Rob said. "The way Aunt Ida helped out was huge to me."

Rob needed support because his body was up against a mountain peak too steep and too high to conquer—Crohn's disease. Eighteen months after his first symptoms, his weight dropped down to a skeleton-like 100 pounds, his life on tenterhooks, and with a diagnosis of Crohn's disease with ulcerative colitis in his hand, Rob knew there was no other option but to submit to having an ileostomy.

He called Aunt Ida and asked her what the pros and cons were for ostomy surgery. Sure, having a stoma and an appliance was no walk in the meadow, she explained, but life would look sunny again. "After speaking with Aunt Ida, I knew what to expect," Rob said. "By then, I was so focused on getting healthy again that I didn't care about the ostomy. I figured I'd deal with the nuts and bolts later. I just wanted to feel well again."

On September 11, 1995, colectoral surgeon Dr. Michael Pezim opened up Rob's abdomen to begin the procedure. What he saw shocked him. The intestine wall had attached itself to Rob's liver, making it appear that Rob had cancer. He knew the young man was dying and didn't have long to live.

Dr. Pezim and the surgical team worked quickly to remove Rob's large intestine and equip him with an ostomy. "When it came down to losing my colon or losing my life, it wasn't a hard decision to make," Rob said.

He didn't gain weight, however, in the early weeks of recovery. In fact, he lost more weight. At one point, he was down to 85 pounds and looked like a Holocaust survivor.

"Actually, I looked more like a starving Ethiopian because of the prednisone," he explained with a wry smile. "My stomach was bloated and extended out, and my face was puffy as well."

So Rob set his very disciplined mind on three simple goals: eating, exercising, and gaining weight. As his body healed from the surgery, his health improved quickly as Rob gradually put some meat on his skin and bones. "I was amazed at the muscle memory and how fast my muscles returned after my body cleared the prednisone and actually began absorbing nutrients again," he said.

At first, dealing with the ostomy appliance went pretty smoothly. A nurse showed him what he needed to do, and Rob reminded himself that this was his new reality, and the sooner he understood that, the sooner he would get used to what he had to deal with.

Yet merely telling himself that he should be able to deal with it didn't seem to make his situation any better. Mentally, Rob felt completely overwhelmed and unprepared for the massive changes surrounding his new body image. He questioned whether this was a peak beyond his abilities. He couldn't seem to summon the mental discipline that had come so easily when he was climbing a sheer face of rock—preparing a route to the top, focusing on the next handgrip, and keeping the final goal in mind. "I was mentally weak, something I didn't fully understand until years later," he confessed. "I wasn't anywhere close to recovering physically, mentally, or spiritually."

Rob says he was severely depressed during those first few months after surgery. Sure, his body had rebounded well, putting on weight and gaining strength quickly. But he couldn't shake off the feelings of malaise.

After several months, when he felt physically up to it, he decided to begin climbing again. But in his still depressed state, he says he started not caring what happened to him. He began taking irrational risks that he had never taken before—like free climbing a hundred feet off the ground without being secured with a rope. This was extremely dangerous because if he lost his grip and fell, there was no way he would survive.

"I guess I was still angry inside and began living a pretty irresponsible lifestyle," he said. "I was climbing hard but taking risks that were daring and kind of stupid—well, really stupid. I took those insane risks not necessarily in the hopes that I'd get killed but because I didn't care what happened. I mean, here I was, free climbing with no ropes, nothing to stop me from falling and killing myself. One time, I had a scary moment and nearly lost it. I remember saying to myself, *'What are you doing out here?'* That focused me a bit," he said.

"I started to train for a triathlon by riding my bike back and forth from Vancouver to Richmond, where I worked. It was a twenty-kilometer ride. While riding home one day, I got hit by a car. I was fortunate that I didn't break any bones, but the accident twisted me up pretty badly. I spent a few weeks doing physical therapy, and it was during that time that I realized that I hadn't mentally recovered from dealing with the Crohn's disease. Even though I had put my weight back on and had gotten stronger physically, I still hadn't dealt with the mental and spiritual side of things. I realized that if I didn't wrestle with those issues, then I wouldn't be completely recovered and couldn't do myself or anyone else any good."

His rock climbing habits kicked in. Like scaling a sheer rock race, Rob knew he had to take his time and remain patient. With an ostomy, that meant he needed to take time to not only heal his physical wounds, but his mental trauma as well. Rob says it took him close to a year before he could talk comfortably about what he had gone through and deal with the reality of living with an ostomy.

When he passed that hurdle, he decided to take some business classes at a nearby college, Capilano University, with the idea of starting a mountaineer guiding company. One of his business classes was right up his alley since it involved leadership training as well as outdoorsy pursuits like ocean kayaking and backcountry runs. It was in class that Rob was given an assignment of writing a business proposal. The students were told to dream big and think through what it would take to accomplish that goal.

An idea started to form in Rob's mind . . . an idea about climbing the tallest mountains on the planet's seven continents. He titled his paper, "Climb the Seven Summits," and he outlined his plan to tackle the seven peaks to raise awareness for those suffering from Crohn's disease. This paper was written in 2001, six years after his surgery.

One of Rob's instructors happened to be a professional climbing and backcountry guide named Brian Jones. He encouraged Rob to do more than write about climbing the Seven Summits but to actually step out and "Just do it," as the Nike ad said.

Rob followed that advice, and within several months, he found himself in the Caucasus Mountains of Russia, part of a mountaineering group climbing Elbrus, the highest peak in Europe at 18,510 feet. He came home energized from his success at climbing his first Seven Summit peak and was ready to tackle the next—Kilimanjaro in Africa.

While preparing for his expedition to Africa, Rob was surfing the Internet one evening and came across a website, www.greatcomebacks.com, a place where stories of comebacks from ostomy surgery were shared. "I was inspired by what I read," he said. "I learned that there were other people like me who weren't content to just *survive* ostomy surgery but who wanted to return to their passion and reach out and encourage others. So I wrote the Great Comebacks website and shared my story.

"A month or so later, I was at the airport in Ethiopia, getting ready to board a flight home after climbing Kilimanjaro when I decided to go online to check my email. To my surprise, I found a note from Rolf Benirschke, who said he had just read my story and thought we should talk. He felt we shared the same desire to be an encouragement to others and believed we might be able to work together some day to raise awareness for Crohn's disease and ostomy surgery. I ran around the airport like a madman just so excited to hear from Rolf. I had read about him and his ostomy surgery and what he had overcome. I had admired him from afar because he had not only returned to kick for the San Diego Chargers in the NFL, but here was the guy who had started this amazing Great Comebacks program. Now he was reaching out to me!"

It wasn't long before Rolf suggested a meeting with Dave Johnson, who was a vice president at ConvaTec (the company that supports the Great Comebacks program). Dave flew out to Vancouver to meet Rob and to discuss how they might work together.

Dave, who has since been promoted to CEO of ConvaTec, was greatly impressed with Rob and his story, along with his burning desire to inspire others. That's when he and Rolf invited Rob to become the first international "Global Ambassador" for the Great Comebacks program.

Rob didn't have to be asked twice. "I didn't know if I was worthy of such an honor," he said, "but I was sure excited to help."

One of the ways they all decided Rob could help was for him to continue his quest to climb the Seven Summits. Aconcagua in Argentina was scaled in January 2004, Mt. McKinley (Denali) was summited in June 2005, Antarctica's Vinson Massif was climbed in January 2006, and Carstensz Pyramid, the tallest peak in Oceania region of the world (which encompasses the Australia and Indonesia), was summited in April 2007.

Back to the Roof of the World

A year later in April 2008, Rob found himself at Everest's Base Camp with his Canadian expedition group. Climbing the world's tallest peak is an expensive undertaking; just the permit alone from the Nepal government costs $10,000. When you add in plane fare, the cost of nearly two months of living expenses, Sherpa guides, kitchen help, oxygen bottles, tents, stoves . . . the cost to climb Everest can easily top $50,000 to $75,000.

Tragically, just days before the attempt, Rob was suddenly hit with an intestinal blockage, apparently brought on by a steady camp diet of foods cooked in grease. "At the camp kitchen, they were frying up patties of some kind of meat and frying up vegetables, and I guess that just took a toll on my body—eating everything cooked in oil. My blockage got so bad that I had to be airlifted to the valley below to seek medical attention.

"I had never had a blockage before, so this caught me completely unawares and hit at the worst possible time. At Base Camp, they were trying to feed us Western foods to keep the Americans and Europeans happy, but the greasy food must've compromised my digestive system. All that work and expense to climb Everest suddenly just went down the drain."

Although deeply disappointed, Rob said his quest to scale Everest is not over. He plans to return to Base Camp and complete the Seven Summits by climbing to the top of Mt. Everest in the spring of 2010. If and when he reaches the top of the world, Rob plans to unfurl a small flag from ConvaTec as an encouragement to the several million people around the world who live with ostomies.

Such an act will fulfill a dream of Rob Hill's to climb Everest not just because "it's there" but to show the entire world that you can come back from life-saving ostomy surgery and do *anything*— including scaling the Earth's Seven Summits.

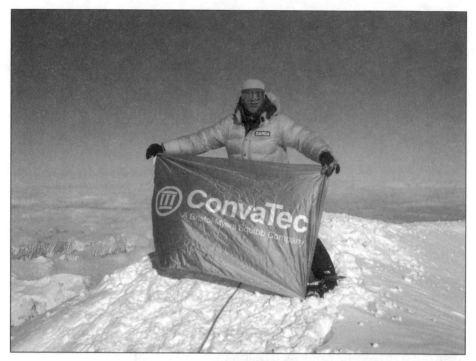

Supported by ConvaTec and encouraged by ostomy patients from around the world, Canadian climber Rob Hill is determined to climb the Seven Summits—the tallest peak on each of the seven continents. The only mountain he has yet to summit is Mt. Everest.

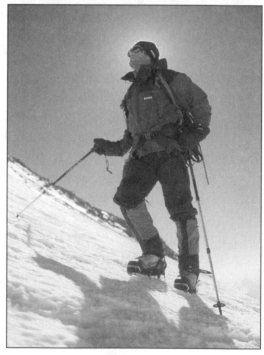

OSTOMY INFORMATION

LIVING WITH AN OSTOMY

When first considering ostomy surgery, many people are concerned that the operation will dramatically alter their lives. Though any surgery should be considered carefully, an ostomy can be the key that opens the door to opportunities locked away by illness. For people who have ulcerative colitis, this operation offers a cure. The following are questions that are most commonly asked by people who are considering ostomy surgery.

What is an ostomy?

There are various types of ostomy surgery, depending on the nature of the illness. A common option for ulcerative colitis is the creation of an ileostomy. The entire colon and, in some cases, the rectum are removed in a one or two-step procedure. The surgeon creates an opening in the abdominal wall, through which the ileum is rerouted to the outside, creating a stoma. To collect stool as it exits the ileum, a disposable pouch is attached to the skin around the stoma with medical adhesive. Since a permanent ostomy is not a cure for Crohn's disease, it is performed only when the disease cannot be controlled medically. Some conditions (e.g., a bowel perforation or abscess) may require a temporary ostomy.

How much time must I allow for daily care?

The maintenance of an ostomy requires only minor modifications in your routine. Daily care consists of emptying the pouch when it becomes one-third to one-half full. You can do this in any bathroom, private or public. This process requires no additional equipment and takes little more time than you previously required to "go to the bathroom." In fact, it may be less time-consuming, especially if diarrhea plagued you before surgery.

Ostomy pouches, like your rectum, have a finite capacity and will overflow or leak if they become too full. Most people report that they need to empty the pouch four to six times a day. You should note the occasions when the stoma is more active (e.g., after meals), and set aside time to empty your pouch. To avoid interrupting sleep, it is helpful to drain the pouch at bedtime, but you may want to empty it again should a full bladder awaken you.

What kinds of pouching systems are available?

Ostomy "appliances" are designed to meet individual needs. There are one-and two-piece systems, pouches with built-in skin barriers, drainable and closed-end pouches, styles offering various depth of convexity, pouches with built-in gas relief valves and filters, and combinations of these features. Years ago, certain types of pouches were designated for specific surgeries (e.g., an ileostomy required a drainable pouching system). Though more options are available today, some ostomies are more difficult to manage than others and require recommendations by healthcare professionals.

How can I find the system that is best for me?

You may want to consult an enterostomal therapy nurse (ETN), a registered nurse who specializes in ostomy care. The ETN will recommend a pouching system and will teach you how to care for the stoma. After your discharge from the hospital, she is available for follow-up care. In time, your pouching needs may change, as normal post-operative stomal swelling diminishes or your weight changes. As your self-reliance grows, you can work with your ETN to select a new system.

How do I care for the skin around the stoma?

Proper attention to the skin around an ileostomy can eliminate painful bouts of raw or reddened skin. Known as "stomal effluent," the stool from an ileostomy usually is liquid and contains enzymes and other digestive acids native to the small intestine. These materials break down the proteins in food, making them easier to absorb. The enzymes, however, cannot distinguish between the proteins they attack and your skin. Thus, if the stomal effluent remains in contact with the skin for too long, painful irritation can result.

People who have ileostomies should never patch a leaking pouch with tape. Change the entire system, and be sure to clean the skin first. Burning or itching under the pouch indicates that some stomal effluent has leaked onto the skin. Pectin-based or hydrocolloid skin barriers always should be used for ileostomy management. They may be used in conjunction with a skin barrier paste. Avoid harsh soaps when cleaning this area. The opening in the pouching system should be accurately sized to prevent the possibility of stool leakage.

Will I require a special diet?

If a particular food bothered you before surgery, it probably will continue to do so. For example, if you suffered from lactose intolerance before surgery, dairy products still may cause diarrhea, bloating, and gas. Some people find, however, that they are able to eat foods that they could not tolerate before.

You may need to avoid high residue or "stringy" foods, such as popcorn and peanuts, because they can cause blockages in the bowel. Don't worry if seeds from cucumbers, tomatoes, or fruits appear whole in your pouch. Even an intact intestinal system will not digest these foods.

If you are unsure about a particular food, try a small portion. If you have no problems, you might try a larger portion next time. Remember, also, that taking time to chew food thoroughly will improve digestion.

People who have ileostomies need to maintain a fluid intake of eight to ten glasses a day or more. To replace potassium and sodium lost in ileostomy effluent, drink such fluids as tea and tomato or fruit juices, in addition to water. Sport drinks such as Gatorade are also excellent for replacing vital electrolytes.

Will the stool in my pouch cause odor?

With proper care, odor need not be a concern. Indeed, you probably have met someone with an ostomy and were unaware of his condition. (Up to 1 million people in North America have ostomies!)

To combat odor, avoid foods that cause gas. You may also use products specifically designed to control pouch odor:

• Pouch deodorizers. These commercially available products, usually liquids, are placed inside the pouch each time it is emptied. The most effective agents attack the odor-causing bacteria, rather than simply mask odor.

• Internal agents, such as chlorophyll tablets or bismuth subgallate. These over-the-counter products are taken orally several times a day, or with meals.

• Room deodorizers. One spray of a concentrated ostomy deodorizer can freshen the air after you empty your pouch.

Can I have a normal sexual relationship?

It's natural to be concerned that an ostomy may alter your ability to function sexually, to feel desirable, and to be the recipient of another's love. But many people find that their sex life improves after ostomy surgery.

Your ability to feel attractive and "sexy" comes from feeling good about yourself. When you are ill, your sex drive may decrease. Perceiving ostomy surgery as a release from illness can help you return to healthy sexual functioning.

In general, an ostomy's impact on your sex life is related to your mind, not your body. Occasionally, however, surgical removal of the rectum can affect a male's ability to have an erection. But this is the exception, not the rule. When careful excision of the rectum is performed, most males retain their ability to have and to maintain an erection.

Discussing your concerns about sexuality with your surgeon or ETN, both before and after surgery, will help you through the initial adjustment period.

Will ostomy surgery affect my ability to have children?

An ostomy provides no barriers to a woman's ability to become pregnant or to have a healthy baby. The only inconvenience may be changes in stomal contour and size during pregnancy, due to increases in abdominal girth. These changes are easily managed by accommodating the pouching system to the fluctuations of the stoma size and shape. A vaginal birth is possible, unless your obstetrician recommends a caesarean section. It's important that your obstetrician consult your surgeon during your pregnancy.

Will an ostomy restrict my physical activity?

Activities, such as jogging, skiing, aerobic exercise, swimming, and even rollerblading, are not contraindicated because of an ostomy. But you will have to avoid vigorous contact sports and heavy lifting. For example, playing football can injure the intestinal tissue from which the stoma is created. Lifting anything heavier than twenty-five pounds can increase intra-abdominal pressure, which can lead to further complications, such as parastomal hernia. This does not mean, however, that you cannot pick up your baby! If work demands heavy lifting or some other strenuous activity, discuss this situation with your surgeon and your employer. Indeed, if you're in doubt about any activity, consult your physician.

Remember, ostomy surgery can give you a new lease on life. Enjoy it!

GWEN B. TURNBULL, R.N., B. SED, C.E.T.N.

SUPPLEMENTAL OSTOMY INFORMATION FROM CONVATEC

ConvaTec is the world's largest manufacture of wound and ostomy care products and has been committed to providing the best products and services to patients since its inception in 1978. For more information, please visit www.convatec.com.

Understanding Your Stoma

A stoma is the opening that has been established in the abdominal wall by your surgery. It is shiny, wet, and red in color, and usually has a round or oval shape that varies in size from person to person.

A stoma does not have nerve endings, so it doesn't transmit pain or other sensations, but it is rich in blood vessels and may bleed slightly if irritated or rubbed. This bleeding is normal, but if it's prolonged or if the discharge from the stoma is bloody, contact your doctor.

After surgery, your stoma may appear swollen. The swelling will diminish, and your stoma will gradually shrink in size. For a few months, you will need to measure your stoma regularly to ensure your pouching system fits correctly.

The skin surrounding the stoma (called the peristomal skin) must be protected from direct contact with discharge. This discharge may be irritating, so each time you change your pouching system, be sure to cleanse this area gently with a mild cleanser that leaves no residue, then rinse with water.

Skin Care

Prevention is an important aspect in maintaining healthy skin and avoiding potential skin problems. Often times, skin problems are caused by leakage of urine or stool onto the skin surrounding the stoma, causing irritation or an infection. Even with the best of care, skin problems can occur. If they do, you and your healthcare provider should seek a solution early because waiting may lead to more serious complications, unnecessary discomfort, and worry.

Healthy Skin

The skin surrounding the stoma should look the same as skin anywhere else on your body. Redness is a sign of skin irritation in people with light skin tone. Lighter- or darker-appearing areas of skin can be a sign of irritation among people with darker skin tone.

You should do your best to protect the skin around the stoma from coming into direct contact with stool. By focusing on a nice secure seal around the stoma, you will have a better chance of avoiding problems.

Be sure to follow these tips:

• Before you apply your pouch, be sure to mold or cut the opening in your skin barrier to the correct size.

• Avoid soaps that contain moisturizers or fragrances as these can interfere with skin barrier adhesion.

• Ostomy skin care accessories can be used to help remove the skin barrier and improve your fit.

• Change your skin barrier as soon as possible if output creeps under the adhesive to avoid having effluent contact your skin.

Activities

Whether you like playing tennis or golf, or enjoy activities such as jogging, swimming, or skiing, you likely won't have to change your lifestyle. With your doctor's permission, you can go back to the same sports and activities you engaged in before your surgery. However, you should avoid heavy lifting and refrain from rough contact sports such as boxing, wrestling, or football without special protection for your stoma.

Clothing

Since modern colostomy pouches are designed to lie flat against your body and aren't noticeable under most clothing, there's no need for a whole new wardrobe. You don't even need special undergarments—pouches can be worn either inside or outside your undergarments, whichever you prefer.

Here are some things to consider:

• If your stoma is at or near the waistline, try to avoid pressure from tight-waisted pants or belts.

• If you want to wear a girdle, make sure it is soft and stretchy.

• Many men who wear athletic supporters find it helpful to wear them one size larger.

• For special occasions and form-fitting clothing, closed-end pouches offer increased security without the higher profile tail closures found on drainable pouches.

• Wearing an opaque pouch may help reduce visibility through clothing.

Intimacy

It's normal to feel sensitive about changes to your body, yet it is important to share your feelings with your spouse or loved one, and to respond to his or her concerns as well.

Here are a few things you can do to help enhance intimacy and enjoy a mutually satisfying relationship:

• It is important for you and your partner to know that sexual relations will not hurt your stoma.

• You may wish to wear a small pouch. There are specialty pouches designed for intimate moments. To learn more, call ConvaTec's customer interaction center at (800) 422-8811.

• If you feel uneasy about your partner seeing your pouch, you can cover it with specially designed underwear, lingerie, or pouch covers.

• You may also want to empty your pouch before beginning sexual relations.

Diet

After recovering from surgery, you can gradually resume eating a balanced diet, unless your physician requires you to follow a special diet. You may wish, however, to avoid certain foods that can cause odor or gas. It's good to remember that if a certain food disagreed with you in the past, chances are that same food will disagree with you after surgery.

Regularity

Just like before your surgery, at times you can experience diarrhea, which can be caused by many things, including viruses, antibiotic therapy, some medications, and your intolerance to certain foods. To reduce diarrhea, eat foods that thicken your stools, such as white rice, applesauce, bananas, creamy peanut butter, yogurt, pasta, and bread. Continued diarrhea can cause dehydration, so increase the amount of fluids and salts in your diet, which will help replenish the electrolytes in your system.

Dehydration

After a colostomy, you no longer have a working colon. This may cause you to lose water and electrolytes. It is necessary for you to drink at least six to eight glasses (or 48-64 ounces) of water or fruit juice each day to prevent dehydration, unless instructed otherwise by your physician.

Signs and symptoms of dehydration:
- dark-colored urine
- decreased urine output
- dry mouth and mucous membranes
- muscle cramps (abdominal or leg)
- nausea and vomiting

Gas

Intestinal gas can be caused by swallowing air, chewing gum, talking while eating, smoking, sipping through a straw, and certain foods. You may wish to avoid foods that cause odor or gas, or are hard to digest. Please ask your healthcare professional about any dietary restrictions that you may have.

Food and beverages that can produce gas:
- beans
- beer
- carbonated beverages
- cucumbers
- dairy products
- mushrooms
- onions
- cabbage family vegetables
- broccoli
- Brussels sprouts
- cabbage
- cauliflower

Foods that can produce odor:
- asparagus
- cheese
- eggs
- fish
- onions
- some spices
- cabbage family vegetables
- broccoli
- Brussels sprouts
- cabbage
- cauliflower

Medications

After ostomy surgery, the way your body digests and absorbs medications may be affected. Make sure to review all of your medications—both over-the-counter and prescription—with your WOC/ET nurse or healthcare provider and your pharmacist.

Some medications can change the color of your stool. You may wish to wear an opaque pouch in order to reduce visibility through clothing.

Some over-the-counter medications/treatments can include:
- antacids
- anti-diarrhcals
- aspirin
- anti-inflammatory agents
- laxatives
- salt substitutes
- sugar substitutes
- vitamins

FACTS ABOUT
INFLAMMATORY BOWEL DISEASE

• Crohn's disease and ulcerative colitis (collectively known as inflammatory bowel disease, or IBD, because their symptoms and complications are similar) are chronic digestive disorders of the small and large intestines.

• It is estimated that two million Americans suffer from IBD, with 30,000 new cases diagnosed in the U.S. each year. New cases per day average 82, or 3.5 an hour.

• Anyone can get IBD, but young adults between the ages of 20 and 40 are most susceptible. (Ten percent, or 200,000, of those afflicted are youngsters under the age of 18.)

• Symptoms range from mild to severe and life-threatening and include any or all of the following:
  · persistent diarrhea
  · abdominal pain or cramps
  · blood passing through the rectum
  · fever and weight loss
  · skin or eye irritations
  · delayed growth and retarded sexual maturation
   in children

• Approximately 20 percent of patients have another family member with IBD, although a specific genetic pattern has not been identified.

• Both the cause of and cure for IBD are unknown.

Treatment

• Medications currently available alleviate inflammation and reduce symptoms but do not provide a cure. The principle drugs used to treat both Crohn's disease and ulcerative colitis are sulvasalazine and corticosteroids.

• A number of new medications, derivatives of corticosteroids and sulfasalazine, are currently awaiting FDA approval. Four such drugs, Asacol®, Rowasa®, Dipentum®, and Pentasa®, have been approved since 1988. Remicade has also been shown to be effective in many patients with Crohn's disease.

• Immunosuppressive agents, such as azathioprine (Imuran®) and 6-murcaptopurine (6-MP), are other medications used to treat IBD, especially in persons who do not respond to more standard treatments.

• IBD is an unpredictable illness—some patients recover after a single attack or are in remission for years; others require frequent hospitalizations and even surgery. Symptoms may vary in nature, frequency, and intensity.

• Without proper treatment, symptoms may worsen considerably and complications may occur.

• Colon cancer may be a serious complication of long-term ulcerative colitis involving the whole colon, even in a patient who is in remission.

Surgery

• Surgery is sometimes recommended when medication can no longer control the symptoms, when there are intestinal obstructions, or when other complications arise.

• An estimated two-thirds to three-quarters of persons with Crohn's disease will have one or more operations in the course of their lifetime. The surgery for Crohn's disease, however, is not considered a permanent cure, because the disease frequently returns elsewhere in the gastrointestinal tract. For ulcerative colitis, surgical removal of the entire colon and rectum (colectomy) is a permanent cure. Approximately 25-40 percent of ulcerative colitis patients will require surgery at some point during their illness.

Emotional Factors

• IBD is not a psychosomatic illness—there is no evidence to suggest that emotions play a causative role. IBD flare-ups may occur, however, during times of emotional or physical stress.'

Diet

• There is no link between eating certain kinds of foods and IBD, but dietary modifications, especially during severe flare-ups, can help reduce disease symptoms and replace lost nutrients.

Effects on the Person with IBD

• The economic and social burden on patients and their families can be enormous. Children and adults must interrupt school and work for repeated hospital stays, and medical and disability insurance often are unavailable.

THE TEN MOST COMMON MYTHS ABOUT CROHN'S DISEASE AND ULCERATIVE COLITIS

MYTH 1: Crohn's disease and ulcerative colitis are caused by stress.

There is no evidence that Crohn's disease and ulcerative colitis are caused by stress. But, as with any chronic illness, symptoms may worsen during a particularly stressful period in a person's life.

MYTH 2: Certain personality types are more prone to develop ulcerative colitis or Crohn's disease.

IBD sufferers were once perceived as people who were emotional or nervous. However, a study conducted by Johns Hopkins University and Medical School concluded that the personality profile of people with IBD does not differ significantly from that of healthy persons.

MYTH 3: Crohn's disease and ulcerative colitis affect primarily older adults.

Anyone can get IBD, but young adults between the ages of 20 and 40 are most susceptible. (Ten percent, or 200,000, of those afflicted are youngsters under the age of 18.) It is estimated that only 5 to 15 percent of IBD patients develop the disease later in life.

MYTH 4: Symptoms can be controlled through diet.

There is no evidence that diet causes IBD. Most people can tolerate a normal diet. In some cases, however, dietary restrictions must be imposed. Some IBD sufferers find that the lactose in milk causes cramps, pain, gas, and diarrhea. Others find a low-fiber diet (avoiding such foods as fruit, vegetables, nuts, bran, and whole grains) helps control symptoms.

MYTH 5: Crohn's disease and ulcerative colitis are "Jewish diseases."

It's true that individuals of Jewish ancestry are two to three times more likely to develop IBD. But researchers know that IBD does not discriminate. Crohn's disease and ulcerative colitis affect persons from every ethnic and racial group, men and women equally.

MYTH 6: African-Americans don't get IBD.

IBD has always been considered more common in whites. However, recent studies show a rising trend among black women.

MYTH 7: Individuals with ulcerative colitis will eventually develop colon cancer.

Under 5 percent of ulcerative colitis patients develop colon cancer. These usually are persons who have had the disease for ten years or more. As a preventative measure, gastroenterologists recommend that patients have a colonoscopy every two years. This exam allows the physician to spot cancer or precancerous changes within the colon.

MYTH 8: Women with IBD have difficulty becoming pregnant.

Women with IBD whose symptoms are under control get pregnant just as easily as women in the general population. Women with active Crohn's disease, however, may have difficulty becoming pregnant until their symptoms are brought under control.

MYTH 9: Many IBD sufferers end up on disability.

While disability may be the only solution in particularly severe cases, most people are able to work and lead productive lives. Indeed, people with IBD are employed in all areas of business and government, at every level.

MYTH 10: People with Crohn's disease and ulcerative colitis cannot live active lives.

Doctors encourage persons with IBD to follow a normal routine. Most people live fulfilling, active lives: they work, raise families, have healthy sex lives, and exercise regularly.

ABOUT THE AUTHORS

Rolf Benirschke, a former placekicker, played his entire ten-year career with the San Diego Chargers from 1977-86. He retired with sixteen team records and as the third-most accurate kicker in NFL history. Rolf received numerous awards during his career, including NFL Man of the Year, Comeback Player of the Year, and he was selected to play in the Pro Bowl in 1982.

Following his retirement, Rolf was the 21st player inducted into the Chargers Hall of Fame, was inducted into the CoSIDA Academic All-America Hall of Fame in July 2004, and was named to the Chargers 40th anniversary all-time team. Today, he is a noted speaker and author and continues his involvement in several businesses in San Diego.

Rolf also remains active with many different charitable organizations in the San Diego community, including the Sharp Healthcare System, the San Diego Zoo, his own Rolf Benirschke Legacy Invitational Golf Tournament, as well as serving as a National Spokesman for the Crohn's & Colitis Foundation of America (CCFA). He is also a longtime supporter of the United Ostomy Association of America and is the founder of the Great Comebacks Program in association with ConvaTec, the largest wound and ostomy care provider in the world.

Rolf and his wife, Mary, recently celebrated their eighteenth wedding anniversary and are the proud parents of four children: Erik, Kari, Timmy, and Ryan. They continue to reside in the San Diego area.

Elaine Minamide, a writer living in Escondido, California, has written for numerous newspapers and magazines. Also providing editorial assistance was Mike Yorkey, who collaborated with Rolf on his first book, *Alive & Kicking*, which has more than 60,000 copies in print. Mike is the author, co-author, and collaborator of more than seventy books. You can find out more about his books by visiting www.mikeyorkey.com.

LOOKING FOR A
POWERFUL MOTIVATIONAL SPEAKER?

Consider bringing Rolf Benirschke and his remarkable story of courage and perseverance and faith as he shares what it took to come back from a near-fatal illness and four major abdominal surgeries to play again the National Football League.

Rolf has been inspiring audiences for nearly thirty years. Groups like Elan Pharmaceutical, Tyco Healthcare, Toshiba, Sports Illustrated, The Hartford, Baxter, Bristol-Myers Squibb, and many others have benefited from his moving presentations.

To learn more about Rolf's speaking availability, please call (858) 259-2092 or e-mail his assistant Barbara Morgan at: barbmorgan@sbcglobal.net. You can also reach him and learn more about his Great Comebacks Program via the Internet at:
www.greatcomebacks.com

**Would You Like to Purchase
Extra Copies of This Book?**

If you would like to purchase additional copies of *Embracing Life* or Rolf's previous books, *Alive & Kicking*, and *Great Comebacks from Ostomy Surgery*, copies are available for $19.95, which includes shipping and handling. Quantity discounts are available.

To contact Rolf, please write:
Rolf Benirschke
Rolf Benirschke Enterprises, Inc.
P.O. Box 231429
Encinitas, CA 92023
(858) 259-2092
barbmorgan@sbcglobal.net